NeanderThin
A Cave Man's Guide to Nutrition

by

Ray Audette

with

Troy Gilchrist

Cover design by **Mark H. Bennett**

ISBN # 0-9646345-1-1, $12 SRP
Copyright March, 1995, 1st ed.
Copyright September, 1995, 2nd ed.
Copyright June, 1996, 3rd ed.

Paleolithic Press
6009 Laurel Oaks
Dallas, Texas 75248

TO:

Grayson Haak Audette
"Who, while just a spirit,
caused this book to be made."

and

Renee E. Solinger
Spiritual inspiration
and
C.P.A.

Acknowledgements

As I am not a doctor or a scientist, I have benefited greatly from many indepth conversations with each of the following people: Dr. Alan S. Brown, Dr. Michael R. Eades, Dr. Vaughn Bryant of Texas A & M University , Dr. S. Boyd Eaton of Emory University and Dr. Loren Cordain of Colorado State University. Without the contributions each made to the research process of which this book is the final product, *NeanderThin* would not have been possible. I am grateful to each for his contribution.

Thanks to Jeff Scroggins for contributing his culinary expertise, recipes and radioactive banjo licks to the project.

Thanks also to Mark Bennett for plugging the book's third edition cover design into 220.

Foreword
by
Alan S. Brown, M. D.

I first met Ray Audette when we were both nine years old. He had just transferred into my fourth grade class and came to my house for his first cub scout meeting. He seemed fascinated by my collections of bird nests, shells, insects and butterflies. When he found out that my father kept a menagerie in the waiting room of his orthodontia clinic, he was hooked. As my after-school chores consisted of caring for this little zoo, Ray appointed himself my assistant and best friend.

Every day after school when other boys played sand-lot sports, Ray and I would feed the animals, clean the fish tanks and collect new specimens from the local ponds and woods to fill the terrariums and aquariums. In between these endeavors we would study nature and conduct experiments. Thus I conducted my first x-ray experiments (the effects of dental x-rays on marigold seeds) and surgery (compound fracture of a pigeon wing) with Ray by my side.

In many ways we were very similar. We both kept falcons. We were both well read for our age (they didn't call us nerds then though they might today). In the summer of the fifth grade I went to a school for gifted children, and Ray went to high school. I took up the clarinet, and Ray took up the violin. I wasn't a good athlete and when we chose sides for sports, Ray was always chosen after me. We were very close for several years. Eventually, Ray moved to Texas to study philosophy, and I remained in New York to begin my medical education. We drifted apart and didn't keep in touch.

I was, therefore, very surprised when, twenty-five years later, I received an overnight package containing the manuscript of this book. I was even more surprised when Ray informed me by phone that the *NeanderThin* program was partially inspired by my own experience with food allergies. Since childhood I have been severely allergic to wheat, corn, soybeans, chocolate, eggs, nuts and fish. According to Ray, my own ability to cope with these dietary restrictions under any circumstances gave him the confidence to give up the staple foods of modern life.

Naturally I read his book immediately. I found it well written and not filled with the usual medical jargon. It's entertaining and in places displays great wit.

More importantly, this work represents a paradigm shift in our views of nutrition and obesity. Ray's view of a natural diet as being the one possible without technology is purely logical. His view of obesity as an immune system response to foods introduced by technology is revolutionary.

Whether the reader is a physician or layperson my professional advice is the same: Take two tablets (see the chapter entitled "Ten Commandments"), and call on your local library to check out Ray's references as I have done. As most of these references are peer-reviewed sources, they contain well-researched and accurate information. Through their own references the articles and books listed in the bibliography also make good starting points for further research.

After seeing your own results and reading the literature, I'm sure you will agree, as I do, with the principles of *NeanderThin*. Happy hunting and gathering!

***

Dr. Alan S. Brown is a physician in Springfield, Massachusetts, where he practices radiology and Paleolithic Nutrition. He received his Bachelor's degree from Clark University in Wooster, Massachusetts, and his Doctor of Medicine degree from the Brown University Program in Medicine. Dr. Brown is also an active member of the American Medical Association and the American Board of Radiology.

Table of Contents:

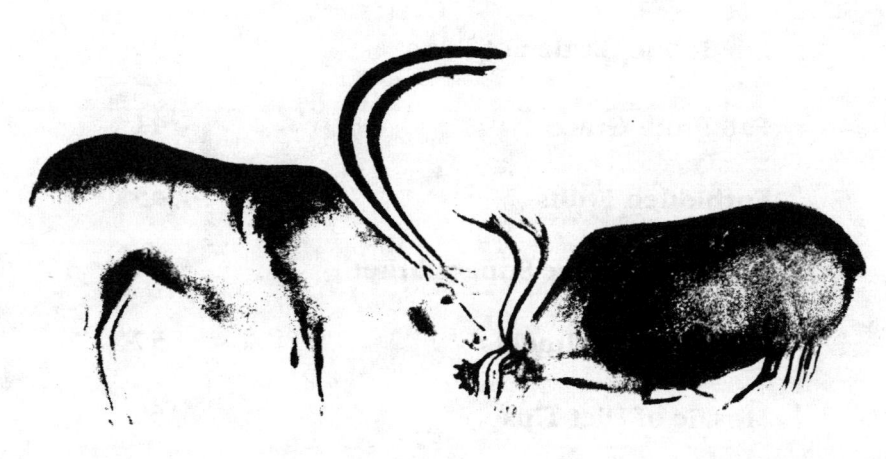

FIRST LAW

Do Not Eat The Fruit Of The Technology[1] That Makes Edible[2] The Inedible[3].
Genesis 2:17

Notes on Translation

[1] English for " Tree of Knowledge " From the Greek *tech* (weave) and *nology* (of knowledge).
[2] In ancient Hebrew synonomous with "good."
[3] In ancient Hebrew synonomous with "evil."

1

Pilgrim's Progress
A History of Dieting

As with any living creatures, humans must be constantly concerned with food. No matter what else occupies our time and efforts, we must eat to survive. Our preoccupation with eating is expressed in the prehistoric record in the forms of tools used in obtaining food and cave art depictions of hunting strategies. Even the most primitive of the preliterate tribes have food taboos in their oral traditions.

Some of the most ancient of writings are the traditional scriptures of the great world religions. In all of these we can find the prohibition or recommendation of many kinds of foods. Dietary rules vary from religion to religion according to the agricultural practices of the geographical regions involved. These philosophies have continued to evolve as problems produced by new technologies made new forms of civilization necessary.

Ancient civilizations were models of economic efficiency. By using simple inventions such as the plow, metalwork and sailing ships, they were able to dominate the known world. Each would fall in turn as they reached the technological limits of both their productivity and their armies.

Our current interest in diet is rooted in the Industrial Revolution and its effects on the diet and lifestyle of 19th-century humans. In the early 19th century people moved from farms to cities to work in the new factories made possible by the invention of steam power. As urban population densities grew feeding the new workers became difficult. These displaced farmers no longer lived where their food was produced, so new methods of food preparation, preservation, transportation and distribution were required.

Inventors and entrepreneurs were quick to rise to the occasion with solutions to the problems of mass food production. Steam-powered mills began to produce white flour, which had a much longer shelf life than previous whole grain products. Bottled food, perfected by Napoleon for his conquests, soon gave way to canned foods using the same techniques. Traditional methods of salting and curing meat were modified to allow mass production. And for the first time chemical preservatives were added to extend the shelf life of foods. With the advent of new processing technologies, food could be mass produced at a central location and transported by newly-invented steam-powered boats and trains to almost any place in the known world. New grocery stores and restaurants were established to sell the new food products wherever people lived.

While the new commercially-produced foods were inexpensive and plentiful, the traditional farm fare of fresh meat, fruits and vegetables did not become affordable or accessible to the average city dweller until the 20th-century invention of refrigeration. Urban populations came to depend on baked goods prepared locally, imported flour, processed meats (salted, cured and canned) and canned or pickled fruits and vegetables. Fresh foods, such as fruit or poultry or fresh ham were reserved for Sundays if you were comfortably middle class or Christmas if you were a worker.

The trend toward manufactured foods was to spread even to the countryside. Farmers found that by eating store-bought foods they could concentrate their resources and efforts on raising fewer crops with a resulting increase in productivity and profits.

Without a revolution in food the Industrial Revolution and the resulting urbanization of even remote towns would not have been possible in such a short period of time. But this change came at the cost of human health.

People began to experience severe digestive problems and increasing obesity in the 1800's. Dyspepsia became one of the most common ailments diagnosed by doctors. Doctors also began to diagnose certain diseases for the first time, including rheumatoid arthritis and multiple sclerosis (MS). Various vitamin deficiencies (pellagra, scurvy, etc.) also became endemic even in rural populations.

Faced with 19th-century doctors' relative disinterest in nutrition, the inventive minds of this period came forward to fill the void of wisdom concerning health and nutrition. Many colorful characters emerged during the 1800's offering cures for the national case of dyspepsia.

One of the first to stress the inseparable connection between diet and health was Sylvester Graham (of Graham cracker fame). Graham advocated a vegetarian diet with an emphasis on whole grains and fresh, raw fruits and vegetables. Through his lectures he became a national figure. And given the unavailability of fresh meat and the deplorable state of meat packing plants during this time, it's no wonder that his program helped many to improve their health.

Weight loss was another problem waiting to be addressed by a talented amateur. In the 1840's an English businessman named William Banting became concerned about his increasing obesity. After consulting with friends and associates, he arrived at what today we would call a low-carbohydrate diet. His subsequent success in reducing his considerable girth led him to write the world's first book on diet and weight loss. Banting's *Letter on Corpulence* was a best seller for several decades .

Acting on a revelation from God in 1863, Sister White, founder of the Seventh Day Adventist Church, led her followers to consume a vegetarian diet that incorporated many of same foods as Graham's diet. Sister White and her husband subsidized the medical education of one of their young followers and helped him establish a health resort in the Adventist hometown of Battle Creek, Michigan. Dr. John Harvey Kellogg opened his sanitarium in 1876.

A proponent of what he called "biologic" living, Kellogg's prescribed treatments of electroshock, light baths, hydrotherapy (baths, saunas, etc.) and 15-gallon yogurt enemas would be considered of questionable value today. Nevertheless, Kellogg's temple of health, called "the San," was considered the most advanced institution of its kind both nationally and internationally.

Ever-increasing numbers of patrons were exposed to a gleaming white facility that closely resembled the health spas of today. Its rooms were filled with newly-invented exercise machines and groups performing calisthenics and laughing exercises. Steam baths, saunas, vapor rooms and swimming facilities were available. Results were measured by the latest testing equipment, which was used to examine muscle development, lung power, body fat and the chemical composition all the body's waste products.

The menu at the San would evoke a sense of *deja vu* in anyone familiar with the USDA's Food Pyramid. Kellogg advocated a low-fat, high-complex-carbohydrate, high-fiber diet. Meat, especially red meat, was to be avoided at all times, and Kellogg's research labs invented several protein substitutes, including many forms of breakfast cereal, peanut butter and soy and yogurt concoctions. These were served to patrons in carefully-measured portions. When the technology for measuring food nutrient composition became available, patrons were provided menus with fat, carbohydrate, protein and fiber quantity listings similar to the labels on today's food packaging.

Although weight loss was not an overwhelming concern of Dr. Kellogg's (he was a very fat man) for his patients who wished to lose weight he recommended reducing calorie and fat consumption, while increasing indigestible fiber intake to encourage frequent defecation (three or four times daily). Combining the San's intensive dietary and exercise programs, many patients achieved significant weight loss. But the difficulty of maintaining the Kellogg regimen led to many repeat visits by inmates of the sanitarium.

Dr. Kellogg wrote over 200 articles and eighty-one books and performed over 22,000 operations before his death in 1943. This impressive body of work, along the Kellogg Foundation established by his brother W. K. Kellogg, provided the basis for contemporary nutritional thinking.

Lulu Hunt, another harbinger of today's common dietary wisdom, used the precise measuring pioneered by Kellogg to introduce a new measure of food value to the overweight public. Published in 1918, her book *Diet and Health With Key to the Calories* recommended the 1200 calorie low-fat, high-carbohydrate diet familiar to even the most casual follower of diets.

Others, however, were following in the footsteps of Banting. In 1888 Salisbury published a diet book that recommended a low-carbohydrate regimen. To make cheap cuts of range-fed Texas beef more palatable he recommended they be ground and mixed with fat. The "Salisbury Steak " lacked only the bun and garnishes of today's hamburger.

Born to Icelandic parents in a frontier town in Canada, Vilhjalmar Stefansson was famous in the earlier part of the 20th century for his Arctic explorations. After a brief career as a cowboy he became an anthropologist and studied at Harvard University. Through Harvard connections he received his first opportunity to go to the Arctic in 1906.

As his first expedition involved a long sea voyage and Stefansson was prone to seasickness, he offered to journey to the base camp in the Canadian Arctic by the overland route. Arriving in the fall at the mouth of the McKenzie River, he was dismayed to learn that the ship carrying the expedition team and supplies had been frozen at sea hundreds of miles away. With only the three-piece suit he had worn on the trip from Cambridge, he had to make plans for the winter. Stefansson's calling as an anthropologist led him to refuse the charity of the few white men in the area; instead, he moved in with an Eskimo family. He lived in their home, adopted their style of clothing, hunted with them and ate their diet.

These lessons would serve Stefansson well in his future career as an Arctic explorer and lecturer. While others explorers depended on tons of stored food and equipment, Stefansson needed only his rifle and the knowledge given him by the natives to probe the northernmost reaches of this unknown world. In expedition after expedition he gained greater and greater fame as the last white man to discover new land in the Americas and meet Eskimo who had no previous contact with civilization.

In between expeditions Stefansson went on lecture tours where, with his strange eating habits, he garnered much attention. Having adopted the Eskimo diet during his 1906 expedition, he saw no reason to give it up. This meant that he never ate vegetables. In the age of Kellogg this was thought to be impossible, so in 1929 Stefansson and a fellow explorer submitted themselves to a one-year scientific study at a New York hospital to determine the effects of an all meat and fat diet on their bodies. Surprisingly to doctors and researchers they thrived on it.

Stefansson maintained his Eskimo diet until he was sixty and married a woman half his age. According to his autobiography, she tempted him with desserts and fancy baking until he began to eat in an almost civilized manner.

After eleven years of this domestic bliss Stefansson suffered a minor stroke in 1960. During his recovery he resumed what he called his Stone Age diet. After an almost complete recovery, he wrote his book *Cancer: Disease of Civlization*, in which he described the lack of what we now know to be autoimmune disorders among primitive, Stone Age peoples discovered by himself and other explorers, missionaries and seafarers throughout history.

During World War II, scientists working for governments on both sides had access to new kinds of lab animals: millions of military conscripts and concentration camp prisoners. By carefully controlling rations and monitoring the results they were able to formulate how to feed people as cheaply (and profitably) as possible. They were also able to determine what vitamins and other supplements were necessary to keep starving people working productively in slave labor factories and on the battlefield.

After the War this data was collected (often for only the price of a one-way ticket to Argentina) and used to formulate many new caloric-reduction diets, as well as vitamin and mineral supplements. New standards for manufactured foods required the addition of supplements to make up for deficiencies inherent to them. The U. S. Department of Agriculture was charged with regulating these new standards and issuing recommendations.

Stefansson experimented with all meat diets during the War while advocating pemmican (a dehydrated and powdered, raw meat and fat dish requiring no refrigeration) as a military ration. His recommendations were never accepted by the U. S. Army (ironically, German Luftwaffe pilots used it in their survival kits). His work did inspire many new low-carbohydrate diets. Some of these in the 50's recommended nothing but meat, fat and water. None, however, were recommended or approved by either the government or the medical establishment. And though all of these diets used the results of Stefansson's work, none included his anthropological slant, which is crucial to understanding how low-carbohydrate diets affect the human body.

R. Buckminster Fuller is famous for inventing the geodesic dome, but most who know of his work are unaware that he advocated a diet of meat, vegetables and fruit. In the 1960's, Bucky found himself very overweight--at five feet, five inches he weighed 200 pounds. Concerned about his increasing size he applied his scientific and philosophic genius to the problem. His solution was, and remains, unique among low-carbohydrate diet advocates.

One of the basic tenets of Bucky Fuller's philosophy is that nature is always most efficient in using energy. The sun is the Earth's main source of energy, and solar energy is directly concentrated in the form of plants through the process of photosynthesis. Theorizing that humans should seek the most energy-concentrated (i.e., the most natural) source of protein and calories, Bucky concluded that he should eat the meat of animals that eat plants.

By applying the unique idea of "energy accounting" to his weight problem, Bucky lost sixty pounds and greatly increased his energy. He continued to eat a low-carbohydrate diet for the rest of his life (he died at age 88).

All of the figures discussed in this chapter can be understood as adherents to one of two philosophies of the human body. The Thermodynamic view of the body sees a machine with parts to be balanced and manipulated. By balancing caloric intake and ouput, by limiting dietary fat and cholesterol, by incorporating synthetic foods and supplements and by advocating strict exercise regimens, Thermodynamic nutritionists strive to create healthy, fit bodies. They treat the body like a steam engine that can be made to run on any kind of fuel with some simple adjustments.

Chaos Theory sees the human body as a biological organism--not a machine. The best example of Chaos Theory is what scientists call the Butterfly Effect: A butterfly flapping its wings in Africa can cause a hurricane in the Caribbean because of the interaction of the components of planetary weather patterns. This interaction can produce results that are unpredictable and disproportionate to the amount of energy expended. Small changes can have global consequences.

Stressing what Chaos theorists call "sensitive dependence on initial conditions," Chaos says that you can never know or account for all the variables involved in the functioning of a system as complex as the human body. Instead of trying reduce fat by limiting dietary fat or correct a vitamin deficiency by adding supplements, a nutritional approach based (consciously or not) on this philosophy stresses the removal of variables (agricultural diet, sedentary lifestyle) that don't match the body's "initial" conditions (naked in the wilderness).

But with all the dietary advice throughout history, as well as the 20th-century tidal wave of health research, how do we know which philosophy is correct? Whose science, whose research should we believe? Perhaps we need a new beginning...

Genesis

I am not a fat person. I have weighed as much as twenty pounds more than my current weight, but even then I was considered thin. *NeanderThin* is not a result of my trying to reduce my weight! *NeanderThin* is the result of my having other diseases which have at their root the same causes as obesity.

More than twenty years ago, while a junior in college, I began to have problems with my joints. I frequently experienced sharp pains in my knees and other joints without traumatic injuries to explain the pain. After a trip to a doctor and several tests, I was informed that I had rheumatoid arthritis. I was told that this was an immune system disease and both the cause and an effective treatment were unknown. It was suggested that I take lots of aspirin and use a cane when the pain became oppressive. I was also told that my condition would worsen in time, and this prediction proved to be painfully accurate.

A dozen years later--still taking lots of aspirin daily and walking with a cane--my career in computers was deteriorating along with my health. My energy seemed to diminish from year to year, which I attributed to the arthritis. I began to experience severe headaches, tingling in my extremities, frequent urination and constant thirst. My energy level was such that I could only work part-time, and I needed frequent naps.

As my bad health was destroying my life, I sought medical advice once again. After consulting with several doctors, it was determined that I was a diabetic and would probably require insulin injections for the rest of my life. As I was only thirty-four at the time, this was a long and terrible prospect. I was also informed that this was an immune system disorder whose cause and cure were unknown.

Needless to say I was very disappointed in both my body's problems and the medical community's inability to deal with them. I decided that I needed to know more about my condition in order to make my life productive once again.

I began my own research project at the public library. I studied the physiology of my conditions as well as the history of both the diseases and their treatments.

From these studies several things became clear: Both arthritis and diabetes are autoimmune system disorders--that is, the body uses its own defenses to attack itself. Both diseases also occur only within agricultural communities. The more recently a population became agricultural, the more likely they were to become diabetic. People like the Inuit and native North Americans who were unlikely to have diabetes when eating their traditional diets, have the highest diabetes rates in the world (up to 80% of their population) when given the agricultural foods of civilization. From skeletal remains it has also been shown that arthritis followed corn as it made its way from Mexico to the rest of the world.

Because these disorders were diet-related and seemed to follow the inception of agriculture, I decided I would modify my diet to emulate that of hunter-gatherers (pre-agricultural or Paleolithic peoples).

Both rheumatoid arthritis and diabetes are immune system disorders. The immune system responds to alien proteins in the human body. Alien proteins are those proteins that in nature would not be found in the human body. Somehow the agricultural diet introduced these alien proteins into our food.

My definition of nature is *the absence of technology.* Technology-dependent foods would never be ingested by a human being in nature. I determined, therefore, to eat only those foods that would be available to me if I were naked of all technology save that of a convenient sharp stick or stone.

Armed only with the sharp stick of my criterion, I headed for the supermarket. Before putting anything into my shopping cart, I thought carefully: Would this food be edible if I happened upon it as it grows in the wild and I had no technology? Of course, during this experiment I carefully tested my blood glucose to see if any improvement occurred.

Expecting only modest results, I was astounded by what actually happened. My blood sugar levels returned to normal almost immediately and remained constant throughout the day. Every day it seemed I had more energy. I slept less than eight hours per day, whereas I had previously required at least ten. Although I lost a few pounds, I seemed to be getting bigger as my muscles became larger and more toned without special exercise. After a few weeks my joints stopped hurting almost completely. Even my ability to think and concentrate seemed to improve. Needless to say, my mood and overall attitude towards life changed for the better as well.

My curiosity was also piqued. Was I the only one to discover this miracle cure? I decided to use some of my newfound energy at the library to find out.

I began to look for similar diets in the medical library. It did not take long to discover that the same diet was first prescribed to cure diabetes in the 1790's. Because the selection of foods was limited at the local market in that time period, the diet was very expensive and thought to be impractical. Why it worked was not understood.

A very similar diet was found to be useful in the treatment of juvenile epilepsy beginning around the turn of the twentieth century. By replacing complex carbohydrates with fats (called a ketogenic diet), great improvements and even cures took place.

It was thought, however, to be impractical and even distasteful and was used only by a few hospitals (most notably Johns Hopkins) as a last resort. Why it worked was never successfully investigated, and it is only recently that many forms of epilepsy have been found to be immune system disorders.

Another variation of this diet was popularized by Dr. Atkins in the early seventies. Millions of people bought his book to lose weight and were successful. An even stricter form was promoted by Dr. Stillman (the Stillman Water Diet). As these diets eliminate large amounts of alien proteins and result in weight loss, could that mean that obesity is also an immune system disorder? To answer this question we must look at what the immune system is designed to do, as well as the known immune system diseases and the characteristics which they share.

The purpose of the immune system is to protect the body from pathogens and parasites that are constantly attacking it. These attackers seek to rob the body of its food and energy and must be overcome in order to insure survival. They include viruses, bacteria, germs, fungi, worms, insects and other types of living things. Because of the number and diversity of attackers, the immune system must have a large number of defensive strategies. As most of these strategies are lethal to the targeted invader, great care must be taken in identifying them as alien and not part of the defending host body or its normal diet.

19

The body detects the presence of invaders by their alien protein structures while recognizing the thousands of proteins that make up the body itself, its diet and beneficial creatures such as the bacteria that live in your gut. When alien proteins are detected, the body can mount any of a number of defensive and offensive responses. Defensive responses include raising body temperature to render the body inhospitable to invaders (fever) or swelling to dilute any toxins that may be present. Offensive responses include providing antibodies that signal white blood cells to attack alien proteins directly. The body may also try to expel the invaders mechanically through frequent defecation (In Latin, *dia - rea*) or frequent urination (in Latin, *dia - betis*).

With all the possible attackers and defenses, a large portion of the body's genetic makeup is the immune system. Indeed, the majority of the DNA coding in every living thing is devoted to the immune system alone. It is not, however, foolproof. Some alien proteins cause the immune system to attack the body itself, resulting in any one of the plethora of immune system diseases which abound in modern civilization.

Diseases of the immune system include arthritis, diabetes, allergies, colitis, Krone's disease, multiple sclerosis, Alzheimer's, endometriosis, many forms of cancer, lupus and most arterial diseases (heart attacks and strokes). The overwhelming majority (95%) of people in developed countries will die of immune system diseases. By contrast, these types of disorders are very rare in wild animals, even when one accounts for natural selection (predators and parasites) removing disabled individuals from their numbers. Among domesticated animals, however, which are fed diets far removed from their natural fare (e.g., American dogs who are fed corn meal--inedible to their canine ancestors--almost exclusively), immune system disorders are again very common. Other diseases which are not traditionally thought of as immune system disorders, such as epilepsy, cavities, myopia, appendicitis, mental illness, attention deficit disorder, chronic fatigue syndrome, acne and emphysema, are also rare in nature.

For this reason, what we call immune system disorders were first grouped together as "diseases of civilization" by the French doctor Stanislas Tanchou in 1843. His monumental paper on this observation led to a 100-year search for "civilized" disorders among primitive peoples by missionaries, whaling ship doctors and explorers who had contact with these vanishing cultures. It was noted that although the native population might be wiped out by infectious disease (smallpox, measles, mumps, etc.) at the outset of their contact with civilization, chronic immune system diseases were unknown to them. It was only when the natives were introduced to the foods of civilization that these disorders appeared and then in direct relationship to the degree of exposure.

Like allergies, other immune system diseases seem to exhibit a threshold of response. That is, until a certain level of exposure is achieved there is seemingly no reaction. One may be exposed to a specific allergen for years with no noticeable reaction and then suddenly develop symptoms. Similarly, a tiny amount of pollen may trigger a hay fever attack if the immune system is already stressed by other allergies that, by themselves, cause no response. All immune system diseases seem to appear suddenly even though the alien proteins that cause them may have been present for years. This type of delayed reaction is necessary to prevent the body from responding to alien proteins that may be transitory or unable to survive in the environment found within the body for very long. By waiting until a threshold level is attained, undue stress is avoided and energy is conserved.

Another characteristic of immune system disorders is that not all people get them when exposed to the same alien proteins. The tendency to respond to a specific protein with an immune system disorder seems to be hereditary. As everyone's immune system is different and the DNA coding for the immune system comprises the majority of the genetic code that one inherits from each parent, humans as a species can carry many more immunities to pathologies and parasites than any single human's DNA could carry. This ensures that some individuals in a population may survive any new parasite, pathogen or plague.

All of these immune system disorder traits are shared by obesity. Obesity is virtually unknown among wild animals. Obesity often manifests as a threshold phenomenon; that is, without changing diet or exercise patterns, a person may become obese. Moreover, no matter what the diet, not all people will become obese. There also seems to be a causal link between obesity and heredity. If your parents are overweight, odds are you will be also.

Looking at people almost anywhere in the world, one is amazed by the number of overweight individuals. These include both young and old and seem to be present in significant numbers wherever people are not facing severe famine.

Many people seek to overcome this problem by reducing the amount of energy available to their bodies through a regimen of caloric restriction or exercise or both. These simple solutions almost never work. The top diet programs all share a very high failure rate. Even people who work out for a living (construction workers, longshoremen, warehousemen, etc.) are prone to be overweight.

Recent studies have also pointed out the contradictions inherent in this method. Poor people, who are most likely to perform manual labor and have little to spend on enticing foods, have the highest obesity rates. The largest long-term nutritional study ever carried out (the Harvard Nutrition Study) showed that overweight people actually eat significantly less than lean persons.

Our current obsession with low-fat diets is also contradicted by many large scale studies. In one such study at Texas Women's College (now Texas Women's University) in the 1950's, it was shown of three experimental diets, the highest in fat produced greater weight loss than the moderate and low fat diets also employed. A recent study published in the *Journal of the American Medical Association* showed that LDL ("bad") cholesterol levels actually rose appreciably (avg. 24%) on a low fat diet among insulin resistant (overweight) individuals.

Obesity is very rare in nature. Unlike many of the animals we see in zoos, overweight wild animals are virtually unknown. This seems to be the case even when unlimited amounts of food are available.

The reasons for this are apparent when we look at the harsh realities of nature. An overweight animal would be slower and more prone to be eaten by predators. An overweight predator would be less successful in catching its prey. Any obese animal would be more prone to disease. All of these factors would mean fewer offspring and a lessening of that species chances for survival.

Obviously, obesity puts an animal on the losing side of the natural selection process. Why then should it be so common in humans, domesticated animals and even the wild animals kept by man in zoos. The reasons are linked by the technologies that separate the artificial world created by man from the natural environment.

These technologies have also produced many other diseases in both man and his domesticated animals that are rarely found under more natural conditions. Such diseases include diabetes, heart disease, cancer, arthritis and many allergies.

Indeed, if we look at the skeletal remains of man prior to 10,000 years ago, before he developed these technologies, we find no evidence of obesity and very little evidence of the plethora of other debilitating conditions we find so common today.

When we look at the remains of humans immediately following the incorporation of civilized technologies during the Neolithic Revolution, we see at once the obesity and diseases common in the modern world. Our Neolithic ancestors' transition from hunter-gathering to farming resulted in a substantial decrease in life span and a six-inch decrease in average height. Paleo-anthropologists find that these characteristics combine to form a convenient yardstick in determining the technology level of the ancient people being studied--the more diseased the population, the greater its technological sophistication.

As we are talking about ancient people, the technologies involved are not those we commonly think of in this world of computers and rockets to the moon, but rather the simple practices of cooking and agriculture used by all people today and in the historic past. These relatively simple technologies

25

have broad implications concerning what humans eat and, subsequently, our overall health.

This book is not meant to be an indictment of technology. In many ways technology has extended and improved our lives dramatically since about 1850 when we started living longer and growing taller (at least in industrial societies). Mathematically, these benefits do not correlate with just the advancements in medical science or improvements in general hygiene, but do correlate more closely with the rate at which new transportation methods such as railroads, steamboats, cars and airplanes improved our diets. In many ways, following the *NeanderThin* diet plan would have been difficult only fifty years ago and nearly impossible 100 years ago.

Just as if we were trying to formulate the ideal diet for a newly discovered zoo animal, we will look at man, his unique physical attributes and ancestral environment, to determine his ideal natural diet. A diet that will satisfy our need for food without compromising our health or waistlines. More importantly, a diet that will allow us to eat as much food as we need to feel satisfied and full.

No special foods will be required for this diet. All that is needed are foods obtainable from almost any supermarket. At no time will any calorie counting or special measuring of portions be employed. Most people will find food preparation greatly simplified.

It sounds very easy, but it's not. Most overweight people will have to give up many of their favorite foods--permanently. Fortunately the cravings for these foods will pass very quickly for those who commit themselves to the program 100% from the very beginning. Any sacrifice will be compensated for by the ability to eat as much as you want, whenever you want. Many will find they are eating more food than ever before and still losing weight.

We hope that by understanding why the foods to be eliminated are detrimental to your health and weight, you will be sufficiently motivated to stay with this nutrition plan until it becomes part of your lifestyle. As we will show, for the majority (at least 99.5%) of human history it was the only life we knew.

Man
As Created By Nature

In order to understand the makeup of our natural diet, it is first necessary to understand what sort of creatures humans are. We must, therefore, compare ourselves to other creatures and determine how our similarities, as well as our unique features, contribute to our success within the environment we were designed to inhabit.

Man is classified by science as a Primate. This order is believed to have evolved from the order Insectivora (insect-eating mammals). This classification includes many other species of animals such as lemurs, monkeys and apes, which in many respects closely resemble ourselves. We share many family traits including an opposable thumb, binocular vision and (with the possible exception of one species of monkey) an omnivorous diet. More than 95% of all primates have a single-chambered stomach incapable of digesting most complex carbohydrates as they occur in nature (in the absence of technology). Of the 200 species of Primates, only the Colobus and Langur monkeys (about ten species) have a multi-chambered stomach and are thus capable of digesting grains and other complex carbohydrates in their natural raw form.

An omnivorous diet is one which includes both animal and vegetable foods. The ratio of meats to vegetable matter varies greatly between individual species of primates. Some, like the tree shrew,

28

subsist almost entirely on insects while others, like the gorilla, get almost 90% of their food from fruits and vegetables. All are, however, designed by nature to maximize the food resources within their environmental niche. Most primates are found within the tropical forest or at its edges. The forest provides a wide variety of fruits, vegetables, insects and small game which compose the diet of arboreal primates.

The earliest remains of humans are found on the African savanna. To see how this primeval grassland appeared, all we need to do is look at any lawn or golf course. Indeed, anthropologists explain our compulsion to install lawns no matter where we find ourselves as a need to recreate the environment for which we were designed and in which we, therefore, feel most comfortable.

Within this savanna environment, man is the only primate (although baboons can be found on its edges). It is very different than the environment favored by most primates. There are few of the trees whose fruit and leaves provide the bulk of food for the creatures of the forest. Life here is dominated by grasses, the creatures who eat the grasses (not including primates, such as humans, with a single-chambered stomach) and the creatures who in turn prey upon these herbivores.

In the process of adapting to a grassland habitat, the human species evolved several physical characteristics unique in the animal kingdom. These adaptations are what separate us from our primate relatives and help to define our specific niche in the ecological system.

Our unique characteristics include a large lopsided brain, bipedalism, eye dominance (resulting in handedness), a lack of fur and a unique variety of sweat glands. None of these physical traits are found in other animals. By determining the evolutionary advantages made possible by these traits, we will develop a better picture of the niche man was created to inhabit.

In nature, brain capacity is related to the types of activities the associated creature engages in most frequently. Predators consistently have proportionately larger brains than herbivores of the same size, because the activity of hunting requires more cognitive functions than simply eating the next leaf. The largest brains of all are usually found in omnivores. Omnivores must eat a much wider range of plant and animal foods to survive and must, therefore, have a greater capacity to develop and store the strategies needed to obtain these foods.

Man, with his proportionately largest of all brains, is capable of obtaining and eating the largest number of other species of plants and animals of any known creature. This trait is invaluable in the savanna where no single group of species produces enough food to sustain humans year round. It also allows humans to outsmart creatures who are faster, bigger or have better senses than ourselves, and to add these species to the available food resources.

A large brain does have disadvantages as well. Because of our large brain size, humans are physically less developed at birth than other animals. As a result our infants require a much longer maturation period than other similar, but smaller-brained, apes and monkeys.

As the brain uses a lot of energy, the body is required to produce larger amounts of energy from food even as the digestive system becomes smaller in relationship to total body size. As a result the evolving hominid could no longer survive on the low-energy-value foods favored by the other smaller-brained, but larger-gutted, great apes.

The disproportionately small human gut is unique among primates. Compared to other primates, humans have a shrunken large intestine and colon. Our relatively small lower gastrointestinal tract inhibits our ability to extract nutrients from calorically-sparse foods (leaves, stems, shoots, bark, etc.) making us more dependent on calorically-dense foods such as meat, fruit and nuts. The shrinking of the hominid colon occurred in a short period of evolutionary time (only a few million years) as is evidenced by the failure of the lymph node attached to the colon to shrink along with the human colon. This lymph node is called the appendix.

Only two other creatures on earth have an appendix: the rabbit and the wombat. Both of these creatures eat calorically-sparse foods but have evolved the habit of passing their food through their digestive tracts twice--that is, they eat their feces. This allows them to derive extra nutrients from their food similar to the way ruminants (cows, goats, sheep) regurgitate their cud to pass it through their digestive systems a second time.

In comparing the gut ratio (large/small intestine) of humans to other primates, the closest ratios are found in Capuchin monkeys and swamp baboons, both of whom eat more meat than any other primates (except humans). But even their gut ratios are far different than ours. The human gut ratio is most comparable to carnivores, particularly the wolf.

Bipedalism, or walking upright, is found only in humans and flightless birds such as the ostrich. Both humans and ostriches realize several important advantages through this mode of locomotion. The first is maximum eye height for body size resulting in a wide range of vision across the broad plains of the savanna they both inhabit. This trait is very useful whether you are looking for food or avoiding predators. The second advantage is the energy efficiency of bipedal locomotion first exploited by the dinosaurs more than 100 million years ago. Whether you are a tyrannosauras rex, a roadrunner or a human, this energy efficiency gives you a tremendous advantage over your four-legged prey. Bipeds are also able to extend their food search over a much wider geographic range.

Because man also has his primate opposable thumb and his hands are free when walking, he can carry objects or food over large distances. This is one of man's most important traits as it allows him to not only use tools as the apes do, but also to carry these tools from place to place and use them for multiple purposes. The ability to carry food also helps overcome the disadvantage of a slowly maturing infant by enabling others to help in gathering food for both mother and child.

Even before hominid brains developed their great size evident in modern humans, they developed a unique shape. All hominid brains exhibit longitudinal asymmetry (lopsidedness). Eye dominance, produced by the unique shape of our brain, produced handedness, which--when combined with our carrying ability--resulted in a new skill unparalleled in any other life form: the ability to throw an object with accuracy. This ability is what has allowed humans to become the most efficient hunters on earth. It has given us the ability to hunt not only small game as the monkeys and apes do, but also to hunt animals much larger than ourselves and much faster than we are. A single human with a sharp stick can kill any other creature on earth--a claim a Bengal tiger would envy.

The final unique physical trait of humans is the combination of our lack of fur and our unique method of sweating. Human sweat is formulated to evaporate very quickly when compared to the sweat of other mammals. We are also capable of sweating a much greater volume of liquid than other creatures. Our bare skin exposes this efficient coolant directly to the wind and sun aiding the evaporation process. The hair on our heads keeps the hot rays of the sun off our heads where we are most prone to overheating. This efficient cooling system allows humans a high level of activity under high temperature conditions which would quickly cause other animals extreme distress.

The equatorial African savanna has a very warm climate year round. During the heat of the midday sun almost all animal activity comes to a halt. Predators hunt during dawn and dusk or at night. Grazing animals move as little as possible in the heat of the midday and seek the few shade trees and wallow holes that are available. Only man is capable of sustained physical activity in all but the very hottest hours of the day. This gives man a window of opportunity for hunting when competition from other predators is scant and prey animals are sluggish.

Using these gifts of evolution, humans developed one of the most diverse diets known in the animal world. A wide variety of fruits, vegetables, nuts and berries could easily be gathered or dug from the ground with simple tools and eaten without further processing. Almost any animal food, including small and large game, could be hunted successfully. All of these foods could be brought back to a central location to be shared with all members of the group. When foraging for vegetable foods or hunting became difficult because of season or overconsumption, humans could easily move themselves and their few tools to a new location without need of domestic draft animals.

Hominids lived this way for over two million years. Today we call this lifestyle hunter-gathering. We were so successful at it that humans were able to expand beyond our original environment to virtually all parts of the world. The period of time when all humans were hunter-gatherers is known as the Paleolithic Era. This era lasted until about 10,000 years ago when the new technologies of agriculture were ushered in during the period known as the Neolithic Era. By examining the lifestyle of Paleolithic man we can come to a better understanding of how these technologies changed our lives and health.

Life In The Garden of Eden

Although hunter-gathering has largely disappeared as a lifestyle in today's world, much is known about how hunter-gatherers lived and ate. By examining the fossil remains of Paleolithic humans (bones, feces and artifacts) and by studying the lives of people such as the African Bushmen and Arctic Inuit (Eskimo), who persisted in hunter-gathering into the 20th century, scientists have a clear picture of how these people lived and died.

Hunter-gatherers lived quite well compared to the way they are often portrayed in contemporary works of fiction. In many ways they enjoyed considerably better conditions than the Neolithic and modern people who followed them.

The search for food among hunter-gatherers has often been thought of as a long and laborious process by those of us who are used to the convenience of supermarkets. Studies of contemporary hunter-gatherers have, however, dispelled this myth conclusively. Among hunter-gatherers living in the harshest desert and Arctic conditions, it has been found that they work less than three hours per day. These hours not only include the time necessary to obtain and prepare food but also the time to provide housing and clothing.

The ease by which food was obtained can be explained by the sheer number of food sources available to man because of his physical traits. Although modern man gets 90% of his calories from just twenty species of plants and animals, a typical Paleolithic hunter-gatherer got his nutrition from over a hundred species. All of these sources were edible raw and required little processing.

Famine is virtually unknown among hunter-gatherers. Drought only serves to make game easier to obtain as the weakened animals cluster at the few remaining water holes. If these dried up, people would simply move to a new area. As man was used to seasonal migrations to follow the game herds and the fruiting of plants, relocation would cause no unusual hardship.

With all of these food sources available, man did not hesitate to eat his fill. Recent studies of contemporary hunter-gatherers have shown that they eat considerably more food every day than the average American. As their food-gathering and other activities burn fewer calories than a leisurely round of golf, we would expect these people to be quite heavy. This is not the case.

These same studies have shown hunter-gatherers to have the lowest fat to total body weight ratio of any people on earth. Hunter-gatherers also show amazing physical fitness and muscle tone when compared to similar agricultural people who work longer and harder every day in the course of their farming activities.

The health of Paleolithic hunter-gatherers was also excellent. Most evidence of early death from this period indicates that the principal causes were infectious disease, trauma and the perils of childbirth. Those who survived these hazards could expect to live as long as we do today. Moreover, those who did survive showed few signs of the chronic tooth decay, osteoporosis, obesity, diabetes, cancer, heart disease and arthritis that plague our older population.

Toward the end of this idyllic era, about 100,000 years ago, severe climatic changes required mankind to alter his lifestyle. The expansion and contraction of the polar ice fields due to several ice ages resulted in an increase in the area of the earth covered by grasslands. In adapting to these much cooler, temperate grasslands, man invented new technologies to cope with low temperature never encountered in his original tropical range. These new technologies included new types of clothing and the use of fire to stay warm.

As man's range extended into this new temperate grassland, he encountered many types of animals that thrived in this environment. Along with mammoths, mastodons, woolly rhinoceri and giant ground sloths, there was an animal that closely resembled man in diet and pack behavior. This creature was the wolf. It would come to follow human tribes to eat their leftovers, just as humans would often chase a wolf pack from a kill to steal its meat. Through the evolutionary process of canine and hominid neoteny (the retention of juvenile traits into adulthood), certain members of wolf packs and human bands would form closer bonds than was usual for the two species. This symbiotic process, commonly known as domestication, would eventually transform wolves into dogs and Neanderthals into modern humans. The resulting mixed packs of dogs and man were able to take game which neither wolves or men alone could subdue. The result of this long process was the spread of mankind and his canine partners into every corner of the world. It also resulted in the extinction of many large animals in a relatively short period of time.

Although these new technologies expanded man's range dramatically, at first they had little effect on man's food gathering and hunting traditions. Animals were now hunted for their fur as well as their meat. Meat could now be preserved by drying and smoking them in racks above the warming fire, techniques that merely supplanted the sun drying preservation of meat that had existed for millennia. The same types of plants that were edible raw continued to provide the vegetable component of our omnivorous diet.

Just before the end of the Paleolithic Era, the new use of fire, along with neotenization of several other animal species (goats, sheep, cows), allowed man to eat many types of plants and animal products (dairy) that, without technological intervention, would not be edible by human beings. With the extinction of megafauna (large ground animals), caused by hunting in tandem with dogs, new food sources were needed. These new food sources would, with the Neolithic Revolution, become the staples of modern diet.

The Fall From Grace

Evidence of abrupt change in the behavior and health of people in certain regions is seen in their remains dating from about 10,000 years ago. These changes were brought about by man's new reliance on technology-dependent foods (fruits of the tree of knowledge) for his sustenance.

At the end of the Paleolithic Era, man learned to cook. Meat that was drying or thawing would become roasted on its surface and people soon began to enjoy this new taste. Some traditional raw vegetable foods were also found to taste better roasted when they were accidentally dropped into the fire.

Soon, plants that had never been eaten before were found to be edible when they were accidentally cooked. Seeds that were on the grasses close to the fire were found to have a new nutlike flavor and to be nutritionally satisfying. Soon grains were added to man's diet. Sometimes when fires were built over certain plants, the previously inedible roots would be found in the ashes to join the new menu as potatoes and yams. Likewise, the seed-pods of certain shrubs became our beans and legumes when their branches were used as fuel for the fire, and they were found to be tasty and filling when roasted.

These new foods, which had not been eaten before this time, never became very prominent in the late Paleolithic diet. Although they were easily stored

41

for long periods of time, carrying them from place to place, as the hunter-gatherer bands moved to follow the seasonal migrations of the herds and the fruiting of plants, was impractical.

It was the invention of agriculture about 10,000 years ago that led to these foods becoming the staples that they are in today's diet. Man found that by planting the seeds of these plants, large harvests of these foods could be obtained. Large amounts of food could then be stored, dried and consumed throughout the year. Because of the need to tend, harvest and protect these crops, man largely abandoned his former seasonal wanderings and settled down into the first permanent settlements.

This new need to preserve foods led to other technologies. Pottery vessels were invented about 6,000 years ago and were used to store the new staples. Soon pots were to join other new inventions such as grinding stones and ovens in new cooking techniques such as boiling and baking. These new implements were to further hinder man's ability to be nomadic by the sheer difficulty of transporting them without domesticated draft animals.

As the areas around permanent settlements quickly became depleted of game and wild vegetable foods, Neolithic settlers became more dependent on crops for the majority of their food. These staples were supplemented by small amounts of meat and, for the first time, milk from domestic animals.

The Neolithic diet had immediate effects on man's health. The skeletons of Neolithic farmers show the effects of improper nutrition. They died younger, were shorter and had many more cavities, as well as fewer teeth, than their immediate hunter-gatherer ancestors. These same remains also show the first evidence of obesity in humans.

The tendency to put on weight was to have another effect on the living conditions of Neolithic peoples. In spite of a much lower life-span, population densities grew dramatically. The tendency of agricultural people to become fat resulted in women becoming pregnant at an earlier age and becoming pregnant again much sooner after giving birth. Studies of contemporary female hunter-gatherers have shown them to reach first menstruation several years later than agricultural women. Hunter-gatherer women average four years between births versus eleven months for agricultural women. As it was no longer necessary to carry infants from place to place, the natural constraints on family size experienced by nomadic hunter-gatherers were no longer in effect.

Obviously, greater populations then required larger crops to sustain them. Soon, methods of agricultural intensification, such as the plow and irrigation were invented to boost yields. As these more intensive methods accelerated the exhaustion of the topsoil and populations continued to grow, new lands for cultivation had to be found. The process of colonization continued until recent

history, until the entire world became agricultural,
polluted, overpopulated and overweight.

Forbidden Fruits

We have seen how humans were designed to eat and how dietary patterns have been changed by technology. In order to eliminate the problems of the modern diet, we must return to the natural diet of our Paleolithic ancestors.

The easiest way to accomplish this goal is simply to imagine oneself stripped of all technology except a sharp stick or rock and eat only those foods that would be edible under these circumstances. When foods are looked at in this light, it becomes very apparent which are natural and which are technology-dependent.

The technology-dependent foods include grains, beans, potatoes, milk and sugar. All of these, when found in the wild in their original state, would be impossible to eat. Without the chemistry we know as cooking or the multi-chambered stomachs found in a few species of Old World monkeys, none of these substances is edible (or obtainable, in the case of milk) to a primate (the order which includes lemurs, tarsiers, monkeys, apes and hominids). The forbidden fruits are the source of 99% of the alien proteins which produce the immune system diseases responsible for 95% of all deaths in America. In order to eat in a Paleolithic manner, it is necessary to eliminate these unnatural food from our diet completely.

45

Complete abstinence from the forbidden fruits is also necessary because of their ability to produce cravings for themselves. These cravings have been found to be very similar to alcohol in their effects on brain chemistry. As an alcoholic cannot tolerate even a small quantity of drink, so the person who eats one potato chip will want many more, even several days later. After a week or so following *NeanderThin*, cravings will diminish considerably, only to return dramatically if any cheating occurs.

Grains include wheat, corn, rice, oats, barley, rye and many other seeds of grasses imported from all over the world. Without milling and long cooking all are inedible. Most of these grains are also mutants and have no natural nutritional equivalent.

Although grains are considered the staff of life in many cultures, all of them are extremely carcinogenic. Corn is considered the number one carcinogen in the American diet. It is responsible for more cancer deaths than all of the pesticides, fungicides, herbicides and other additives that contaminate our food. Many scientists believe that corn is responsible for more cancer deaths in America than cigarettes. Grains, in general, are so carcinogenic that the EPA now requires people who are exposed to them in their work (mill workers, grain elevator operators and some bakers) to wear respirators to provide protection against the cancers and lung disease that plague them.

Grains are found in many more products than the expected breads and breakfast cereals. Often they are used as fillers or thickeners in other foods. Extracts from grains such as corn oil, corn syrup, maltose and others are also used to add fat or sweetness to a wide variety of processed products.

Beans are defined as seeds of legume plants, but the term bean is often used in reference to berries and nuts that are also inedible raw (e.g., coffee beans, cashews). Many beans are extremely toxic if consumed raw, such as limas and soy, while others can only be safely consumed raw for a few days during their immature state (e.g., green beans). Some, such as peas and peanuts, are not considered beans in our culture.

The toxins that protect these seeds from creatures that would eat them are only partially broken down by cooking. The remaining toxins in our bean dishes result in the flatulence experienced by many who eat them. In India the toxin residue in a particular type of pea eaten by the poor causes a disease closely related to Alzheimer's.

Extracts from beans also find wide use in processed foods. Soy proteins are often added as a meat substitute, and peanut oil is used as a cheap source of fat in many products.

Most people are familiar with the poisons found in the eye of potatoes. Most, however, are unaware that these same toxins are found in the entire potato and are unaffected by cooking. A staple diet of potatoes also leads to severe vitamin A deficiencies, which leads to blindness in children in many parts of the world. Because of the prevalence of fungal breakouts in cultivated potatoes, they must be treated with large amounts of fungicide, making potatoes the most chemically contaminated food you can buy in America. In some areas, chemical-free organic potatoes are available, but these are even more dangerous because the fungus is far more carcinogenic than the fungicide and insecticides in the supermarket variety.

The practice of drinking milk or consuming milk products of other creatures has no parallel in nature. Although humans, like all mammals, consume the milk their mothers produce during lactation, human milk is quite different in composition from the milk of cud-chewing animals for sale on the grocer's shelf. The milk of herbivores is designed for an entirely different sort of digestive system and often conflicts with that of humans. Many people are lactose intolerant or are intolerant to the acids produced as a byproduct of milk digestion. This also limits the amount of calcium available from milk as much calcium is used by the body to combat the effects of this acidity. Milk drinkers worldwide have very high rates of both stomach ulcers and osteoporosis.

Another effect of milk on human digestion can be shown by comparing the digestion of milk to the manufacture of common white glue. This household glue is produced by exposing milk to acid and draining off excess fluid--a process very similar to human digestion. Indeed the hunter-gatherer will notice that dairy consumption results in a very gluey consistency in what comes out the other end. This stickiness may result in constipation and flatulence.

Milk, cheese and butter also contain very high levels of fat. By eliminating these products altogether, many people will actually lower their fat intake in spite of consuming more meat. Low-fat dairy products have less fat, but the increased levels of foreign proteins and sugars that result are the true culprits--not the fat. As a consequence, low-fat milk-- a staple of obese Americans--actually inhibits weight loss to a greater extent than does whole milk.

Sugar was rarely consumed by Paleolithic man. Without fire and cooking pots to boil saps into syrups, or smudge fires to pacify bees in order to obtain honey, even these primitive forms of sugar were denied to him. The refined sugars that we gobble by the ton were unknown until very recently.

Care must be taken not to replace sugar with other foods that are more natural but contain almost as much sugar as refined products. These include dried fruits and dried berries (especially raisins). They can be consumed if the amount consumed does not exceed the amount of fresh fruit of the same kind that would ordinarily be consumed. One small box of raisins would equal a rather substantial bunch of grapes. Similarly two dried pear halves equal one whole pear.

The five categories of forbidden fruit do not contain all of the fruits of technology. Others include certain gourds (squashes) and even a few nuts which are inedible raw. When in doubt about any food, apply the basic principle of Paleolithic nutrition: Would this be edible when found in its natural state and without technology? If the food in question passes this test it may be eaten without fear and in unlimited quantities.

Alcohol is not to be consumed in any amount from any source. Apart from its obvious damage to the stomach, kidneys and liver, this byproduct of yeast digestion (the yeast equivalent of urine) is well known to put on fat. In Japan, the fattest, most marbled beef comes from cattle fed almost nothing but beer. Alcohol will also produce intense cravings for both itself and other complex carbohydrates, making it almost impossible to follow the hunter-gatherer lifestyle.

As you can see, we have eliminated much of what a typical person eats every day. Because an animal body cannot require that which in nature it cannot acquire, no essential nutrients will be omitted by following this diet plan. As the forbidden fruits are found in most processed foods, consumption of such foods and their associated preservatives, pesticides, flavor and color enhancers, and other chemicals will be largely eliminated.

Manna From The Supermarket

In spite of large geographic areas of the supermarket being off-limits to the urban hunter-gatherer, much of the food there is still fit for consumption. The foods found in a modern supermarket are unsurpassed in variety by those of any other culture since the Neolithic Revolution.

This variety is crucial to the hunter-gatherer lifestyle. By keeping our diet as varied as possible, we assure ourselves acquisition of all of the necessary nutrients, vitamins, minerals and fiber we need for proper nutrition and energy production. By constantly seeking out new foods that fit within our criteria, we will stimulate our tastes and satisfy our need for new food experiences. We will also be following our Paleolithic ancestors who ate a much greater variety of foods than most modern people.

Meat is an important part of any healthy diet fed to a primate. Recent zoo studies have shown that monkeys fail to thrive or reproduce successfully when denied animal protein. For several thousand years man has, through technological progress in the chemical manipulation and combining of vegetable proteins, sought to eliminate the need for meat in the human diet. Despite these technological advances, modern vegetarians still experience the symptoms displayed by meat-starved captive monkeys. As these schemes to provide complete protein often depend on grains and beans, many of these vegetarians also begin to bear a striking resemblance to the Buddha,

51

considered by many vegetarians to be the ideal human form.

Nearly all primates get their animal protein from insects and other invertebrates, eggs, amphibians, reptiles, birds and small mammals. Humans share these tastes, but because of our unique physical features we can also hunt and consume larger game. Our digestive systems have developed along with these features to enable us to utilize these food sources very efficiently. Raw red meat is thought by many scientists to be the most complete source of nutrients for the human body. It is perhaps the only single food capable of sustaining healthy human life when eaten exclusively, as is done by the Inuit (Eskimo) who eat little else during most of the year.

Other aboriginal Americans and explorers ate an exclusively raw meat diet in the form of *pemmican*. This high-energy food is produced by mixing extremely dried and powdered raw lean meat and hard animal fat in a one to one ratio. Pemmican is eighty percent fat by calories, will keep for decades without refrigeration and can sustain a person without vitamin deficiency (scurvy, beri beri, etc.) indefinitely. It provides those who eat it with very high energy from very little consumption (1/2 to 1 1/2 pounds per day if eaten exclusively). Very little waste results as well (1/6 normal solid waste). The benefits of pemmican and other native foods so impressed the polar explorer Vilhjalmur Stefansson that he adopted the Inuit diet in his early twenties and kept to it nearly his entire life (he died at age 83).

Although all meat is edible raw, it is not recommended that supermarket meat be eaten this way. Proper care must be taken to cook or dry such meat carefully to eliminate all bacterial contamination, which may cause food poisoning. Any of the vitamins destroyed during this process are easily replaced by eating fruits and vegetables.

The fat found in red meat is also an important component in the human diet. Without the high levels of glucose (blood sugar) produced by eating the forbidden fruits of technology, the body lacks energy for sustained exertion. Fat provides this source of energy by breaking down into glucose. Because this breakdown occurs only as needed, the body avoids the effects of high levels of blood sugar (diabetes), as well as extreme fluctuations in the sugar level (hypoglycemia).

Although some hunter-gatherers such as the Inuit eat considerably more fat than any Americans, they enjoy the lowest incidence of heart disease among all peoples. Many would attempt to explain this phenomenon as a genetically acquired trait, but this seeming immunity disappears when the Inuit abandon their traditional diet in favor of a civilized agricultural diet (which is much lower in fat and cholesterol). It is easy to understand why when we realize that arteriosclerosis is indicated by high blood cholesterol levels.

Cholesterol is produced by the liver in response to insulin which, in turn, is produced by the pancreas in response to glucose. Cholesterol is used by the body to repair the damage done by excessive glucose to arterial walls and capillaries. Indeed, the highest rates of heart disease occur among those suffering from diabetes (excessively high glucose). Many of the other symptoms of diabetes are also caused by the damage done by glucose to the capillaries.

The urban hunter-gatherer may actually find that he is eating less saturated fat than before. The absence of milk fat and hydrogenated vegetable oils will compensate for any increases in red meat consumption. Because the body must now draw on this fat for energy, less of it will remain in the body for long periods of time. As time passes, the body will produce more of the enzymes needed to utilize fat resulting in more efficient use of both dietary fat and excess body fat. In this way weight loss, if necessary, is maximized.

Other sources of meat include poultry, fish and small mammals, such as rabbits and squirrels. Invertebrates such as shellfish and crustaceans are also good sources of protein and minerals. They cannot, however, be used to eliminate all red meat as this will result in a substantial loss of energy due to lack of fat. The Inuit call this condition "rabbit starvation". They found that if a person only ate low fat meats, such as rabbit, they would starve to death no matter how much they consumed. In the absence of complex-carbohydrates, fat is vital to human nutrition and well being.

Unlike the Inuit, most hunter-gatherers obtain a large portion of their food from vegetable foods. This consists of the leaves, stems and roots of plants that are edible raw as well as fruits, nuts and berries.

Vegetables--consisting of edible leaves, stems, and roots--include lettuce, cabbage, spinach, celery, asparagus, onions, leeks, carrots, radishes, broccoli, cauliflower, edible mushrooms and most herbs and spices. All of these are edible raw and will provide the most nutrition when eaten raw by themselves or when combined into salads. They are only slightly less nutritious when cooked and can be used in soups, poultry stuffing and as a hot side dish.

Fruits include apples, peaches, pears, plums, apricots, avocados, bananas, melons, tomatoes, grapes, dates, figs, olives, citrus fruits, cherries and many more varieties from all over the world. Most are now available year round thanks to modern transportation systems. All are edible raw and should be consumed when fresh, although dried fruits can be used as a convenient snack food if care is taken not to consume more than would be consumed in fresh form. Canned fruits, candied fruits, preserves, jellies and jams should be avoided at all times as most contain very high amounts of sugar and have lost most of their nutritional value during processing.

Nuts are the seeds of trees and include walnuts, pecans, almonds, Brazil nuts, macadamias, acorns, chestnuts, hickory nuts and many other varieties. They do not include peanuts and cashews which are actually beans and are not easily digested in their raw form. Although roasted nuts are available, the hunter-gatherer should consume them in their raw form whenever possible.

Ten Commandments

NEVER EAT:

I. **GRAINS** corn, wheat, barley, rye, rice, oats and all products made from them.

II. **BEANS** all varieties of hard beans, lima beans, green beans, wax beans, peas, peanuts, chocolate, soy and all of the products made from them.

III. **POTATOES** all varieties of potatoes and yams, beets, taro, cassava (tapioca), turnips and the products made from them.

IV. **DAIRY** milk, cheese, yogurt, whey, butter and all of the products made from them--no matter what kind of animal milk was used to produce them.

V. **SUGAR** fructose, sucrose, maltose, dextrose, lactose, corn sweeteners, honey, molasses and the products made from them.

DO EAT:

I. **MEATS**   beef, veal, lamb, pork, venison, chicken, turkey, duck, pheasant, quail, rabbit, all fish and any other form of meat or meat byproduct such as lard.

II. **FRUITS**   apples, cherries, pears, peaches, melons, cucumbers, tomatoes, bananas, avocados, plums, citrus fruits, olives, figs, dates, mangos, kiwi, star fruit, pineapple, plums, pomegranates, passion fruit or any other fruit eaten fresh whenever possible.

III. **VEGETABLES**   lettuce, cabbage, kohlrabi, kale, rhubarb, cauliflower, flowers, broccoli, asparagus, parsley, herbs, spinach, celery, carrots, onions, mushrooms, greens and any other part of a plant that is edible raw.

IV. **NUTS**   almonds, walnuts, pecans, Brazil, acorns, hickory nuts, filberts, macadamia and any others that are edible raw.

V. **BERRIES**   grapes, blueberries, raspberries, blackberries, boysenberries, strawberries and any others edible raw.

A Mosaic of Diet Tips

Many challenges face a hunter-gatherer living in the midst of an agricultural society. As was previously stated, modern transportation makes possible a diet with great variety, so you should not feel that you will be limited in your choice of foods within the guidelines of the *NeanderThin* diet. Even though you might be giving up a great many favorite foods, keep in mind the benefits of eating only food you are designed to eat, as well as the fact that on this diet you can eat as much as you want of those foods which are acceptable. Just think! All you can eat-- and you don't have to watch your waistline!

Being a modern hunter-gatherer is really quite simple in this land of grocery stores and cafeterias. But it does require that you rethink your approach to everyday eating. There can be no more wolfing down of burgers and fries on the way to a meeting. Take-out Chinese is no longer an option. So here are some tips concerning how to go about your hunting and gathering in a successful fashion:

You *can* do this. *NeanderThin* may seem to be a difficult program to practice, but in reality it's very easy. Even the most undisciplined people (Ray, for example) can follow this plan if they can get through the first week without cheating. This book will tell you everything you need to know to ensure your success. And by following up with your own research you will be further convinced of the validity of the *NeanderThin* program. Whether you are slim and in good health or ill and overweight, the benefits you will experience in just a few weeks will give you the resolve to make *NeanderThin* a permanent part of your lifestyle.

Clean out your refrigerator and pantry. Get rid of any foods in your home which are no longer acceptable. Donate any packaged goods to a local food bank if you wish. By removing all "forbidden fruits" from your kitchen, you simplify the task of breaking old habits by removing any possible source of temptation. (Don't forget condiments!)

Understand why you are giving up the "forbidden fruits." You don't have to be a medical doctor or a scientist to understand the physiological reasoning behind the Paleolithic diet. The scientific arguments for adopting this diet are provided in layperson's terms in the earlier chapters of this book. Make sure you understand them. Go to your local library, and do your own research using the bibliography at the end of this book. Not only will you then be better able to explain why you do not want the baked potato that comes with your steak, you will understand why the diet works, as well as how you stand to benefit from it. This understanding will make it much easier to stick with the diet.

Share the hunter-gatherer lifestyle with your spouse or a friend. Upon making the decision to adopt the hunter-gatherer way of eating and living, you may find it difficult to not give in to temptations when they arise. When everyone else at the party is drinking or having cake, you may feel isolated, like you are missing out. By sharing your new way of eating and looking at the world with those who are close to you, you can create a base of support which will make it easier to stick to the diet. You will also be helping others to see the benefits of being a modern hunter-gatherer, possibly convincing those whom you care about to adopt a healthier diet and outlook on the world in general.

Water. The human body is approximately 70% water. It cannot be stressed enough that you should try to consume as much pure water as is possible. Water is essential for the elimination of waste and other body processes. To this end, make sure that you always have ready access to a source of purified water. If you are thirsty and only chlorinated water is available, then drink it. It is better to drink than to go thirsty, but stick to purified water as much as possible. Use purified water for teas or any cooking that may require water; not only is it healthier, but it will improve taste as well. When eating, however, try to limit the amount of liquid consumed as too much may disrupt the digestion of food.

Fat consumption. A common mistake made by neophyte hunter-gatherers is trying to limit fat intake. This will only result in extreme hunger and fatigue and will actually slow weight loss by lowering metabolism. If you have a high-energy day planned, have more bacon (uncured) at breakfast. If you feel drained during the day, use a high-fat snack such as nuts or pemmican to boost your energy. As your body adapts to the *NeanderThin* routine, fat will become more attractive to your taste. Feel free to indulge this new taste whenever possible (being careful, of course, to avoid fats that are not on the diet-- i.e., oils and fats derived from beans, grains and milk).

The Arctic explorer Stefansson learned firsthand of the effects of fat deprivation combined with a low-carbohydrate diet. He detailed a condition resulting from such a diet saying,

> "if you are transferred suddenly from a diet normal in
> fat to one consisting wholly of ...[lean meat] you eat
> bigger and bigger meals for the first few days until
> at the end of about a week you are eating in pounds
> three or four times as much as you were at the beg-
> inning of the week. By that time you are showing
> signs of both starvation and protein poisoning.
> You eat numerous meals; you feel hungry at the
> end of each; you are in discomfort through dis--
> tension of the stomach with much food and you
> begin to feel a vague restlessness. Diarrhoea will
> start in from a week to 10 days and will not be
> relieved unless you secure fat. Death will result
> after several weeks." (Speth, 1989).

Increase physical activity. One of the chief pitfalls of modern life is the tendency towards being sedentary. The effect of such a lifestyle is a degeneration of the body's ability to meet physical demands placed upon it. After a period of time (determined by your physical condition upon adopting the hunter-gatherer diet), your body will adjust to its natural weight, body composition and metabolism. To keep your muscles and bones strong, regular involvement in physical activity is necessary. This does not mean that you have to adopt a rigorous exercise program (unless you so desire). All that is necessary is regular exercise of some kind. This may mean simply adding more activity to daily events: parking further from the store than usual or taking the stairs instead of the elevator. The primary activity of hunting and gathering is walking and observing--learn to do both at once. True hunter-gatherers are light on their feet and aware of their environment. In this respect, the best physical activities are the ones that allow you to develop a stronger awareness of and relationship with your world. Activities such as picking berries, birdwatching, hunting and foraging for mushrooms or wild herbs require that you be "tuned in" to your environment. You cannot just don a set of headphones and forget about the rest of the world. Although health clubs and gyms certainly are avenues to fitness, the best exercise is the kind for which you do not have to change your clothes.

Working out. Bodybuilders and professional wrestlers have, since the 60's, used high-fat, high-protein diets to achieve maximum muscle gain with a minimum increase in body fat. If your goal is to build muscles, *NeanderThin* combined with weight training will greatly accelerate the process. The resulting increase in muscle bulk will increase your metabolic rate whether or not you engage in regular aerobic exercise. The reason to exercise aerobically is not for weight loss but to improve your cardiovascular stamina. Even if you never have to wrestle a sabertooth tiger, as a hunter-gatherer you will find your increased musculature and stamina beneficial in your everyday life.

Sunlight. The common admonitions of the medical community to avoid sunlight exposure should be taken with a grain of salt. Sunlight provides the basis for organic life on earth. The photosynthetic process in plants is totally dependent upon sunlight, and plants constitute the collective lungs of humanity. As such, we are dependent upon the sun for our every breath. Sunlight also provides us with vitamin D, which is essential to human life. As was presented earlier, man is designed to be active during daylight hours. Provided by nature with an onboard air-conditioning system (the ability to sweat profusely), he can keep from overheating even while engaged in strenuous activities during the hottest hours of the day. So do not be afraid to go out in the sun. Overexposure should be avoided of course, but, depending upon your skin type, a certain amount of daily exposure to the sun is completely natural and is to be welcomed--not avoided.

On the road. Traveling should provide no inescapable problems for the foresighted and resourceful hunter-gatherer. If you know that you will be going to a place where it will be difficult to find hunter-gatherer fare, then plan on taking some trail mix (nuts and dried fruit), beef jerky, pemmican or any other such convenient foods. No matter where you are, you can almost always find a restaurant which serves bacon and eggs or a salad and a steak. (Don't forget to carry a bottle of water.)

Pemmican. The hunter-gatherer's miracle food, eating pemmican makes practicing the *NeanderThin* program easy. If eaten exclusively, a small amount per day (3/4 pound for the average adult) will sustain you indefinitely without vitamin or mineral deficiencies. It provides quick energy without filling your stomach. It's easy to digest (95% absorbed in digestion) and produces almost no waste. Since the digestion of pemmican requires no intestinal flora, eating pemmican exclusively for several days will greatly reduce bacterial presence in the gut. If an exclusive pemmican diet is continued for several weeks, the need to defecate will be reduced to one normal bowel movement per week. As such pemmican is an excellent first solid food for infants, and a good choice for anyone suffering from a gastrointestinal disorder.

Invented by North American Indians and used for centuries by French-Canadian fur traders, pemmican consists of equal parts raw, dehydrated, powdered red meat and tallow (animal fat). Building on these basic ingredients, you can customize pemmican to your taste, including spices, nuts, dried berries, etc.

Pemmican is easy to carry (it's highly concentrated), requires no refrigeration or preservatives and provides quick energy--perfect when you don't have enough time to eat. It's also the perfect workout food for the *NeanderThin* athlete who can't carbo-load.

The taste may be unfamiliar at first, but most people who try it eventually find themselves craving it.

"You mean you don't eat bread?" To most people the idea that bread, corn and potatoes should not be eaten is unfathomable. Everything that is said today about nutrition would lead us to believe that our diets should consist of lots of complex carbohydrates and little fat. So telling people that you do not eat grains, beans, potatoes, sugar and dairy products is likely to make you appear a bit strange. Be aware that to see why technology-dependent foods are not fit for human consumption requires a paradigm shift in your viewpoint on nature, nutrition and health. The *NeanderThin* program turns upside down the common wisdom concerning what humans should eat to be fit, trim and healthy. As was previously stated, it is helpful to gain a basic understanding of the scientific evidence that supports the hunter-gatherer diet. This will help you to explain to people concisely in layperson's terms why a diet seemingly high in animal fat will not clog your arteries or give you cancer. If you wish to avoid such discussions, just tell people that you are unable to digest the forbidden fruits and that they make you sick. (Chances are that you will not be lying if you have been following the *NeanderThin* program for any length of time.)

Eating out. At first it might seem that most restaurants are off limits to the urban hunter-gatherer. To be sure, you will find yourself at

66

a loss when trying to order from the menu at your typical hamburger-and-fries joint. Most fast food restaurants will be useless to you. Many use hydrogenated vegetable oil--a highly toxic substance which you should definitely avoid--for cooking. Italian and Oriental restaurants may also prove difficult. Cafeterias, organic restaurants, steak and barbecue houses, and sea food restaurants are all good bets. Most Mexican restaurants serve fajitas, which can be eaten without the tortillas. And most dining establishments will have a selection of salads from which to choose. If you will be eating out with friends somewhere that you may find it difficult to remain on the diet, eat something before you go and order a salad at the restaurant--without dressing, cheese or croutons of course. Also, do not hesitate to customize an order or ask for substitutions. After all, you are the customer and the restaurant staff is there to serve you. As a hunter-gatherer, eating out may cost more than usual, but the money that you will save on doctor bills, medicine and a new wardrobe every six months (to accommodate your increasing girth) will more than compensate.

Snacking. The *NeanderThin* rule concerning snacking is very simple: If you are hungry, then eat. Eat as much as it takes to satisfy your hunger. With this rule in mind, keep plenty of fruit and sliced veggies around. A big bowl of trail mix is definitely invaluable. Cold roast beef, a handful of nuts or small amounts of dried fruit also make for satisfying nibbling. Just be sure that your snack foods are within the dietary guidelines--could I eat this if I were naked with a sharp stick on the savanna? An occasional bag of potato chips or cookies may seem harmless, but nothing will serve better to sabotage your efforts than intermittent carbohydrate infusions.

Read labels. In the course of switching to a diet not based on technology-dependent foods, your reliance on packaged foods will be greatly diminished. In the event that you continue to buy boxed or canned foods, read labels to make sure that the foods contain no grain byproducts (e.g., rice syrup, high fructose corn syrup, corn starch, etc.), bean byproducts (e.g., soy, soy protein, soy sauce, peanut oil, etc.) or added sugars (e.g., sucrose, fructose, maltose, dextrose, lactose, artificial sweeteners, etc.). Remember also that the ingredients will be listed in order from greatest to least amount present in the product. In other words, a product with soy as the fifth ingredient is less troublesome than a product with soy as the first or second ingredient. Of course, you will also want to avoid any food that is treated with chemical preservatives, additives or food coloring agents. Hydrogenated vegetable oil, an ingredient used to improve the consistency and taste of many processed foods, is an incredibly carcinogenic substance and should be avoided, more so than even synthetic chemicals. Shopping at health-oriented establishments will simplify your search for pure foods and make it much easier to find organic sources of the meats and produce which will constitute the majority of your diet.

Detoxify your living environment. Although the focus of this book is cleansing your inner environment of foreign proteins introduced through improper diet, there are many things that you can do to improve the conditions of your immediate external environment as well. Man is not designed to live in a sealed box for seventy years, so keep your house clean and filled with fresh air. Install a HEPA air filtration system if you can afford one. Also, try to use fewer industrial cleaners in your home, switching to natural or "organic" cleansing agents available at most health food stores. Buy a water purification system for your home, and avoid contact with soaps and other hygienic products made with synthetic chemicals. There are many books available on detoxifying your home. Educate yourself and take action to make your living and working environments as toxin-free as possible.

Sweets. Giving up sweets may be one of the hardest things for many people who would attempt to abide by the guidelines of the *NeanderThin* diet. To make up for the loss of chocolate cake and apple pie, try frozen fruit juice or fruit salads. Frozen berries also make a delicious dessert. A fruit smoothie made in a blender with ice, bananas and other fresh fruits, is a good substitute for a milkshake. And frozen bananas taste similar to ice cream. Honey, if used at all, should be used sparingly--no more than a few drops in your tea as a sweetener. In time, your sensitivity to natural sugar will increase to the point that fruit will totally satisfy any desire for sweets that you may have. Not only will cravings for chocolate and candy

69

disappear, should you try to eat such "forbidden fruits" you will probably find that the extraordinary amounts of refined sugar they contain are too much for the newly developed sensitivity of your taste buds.

Fruits are certainly acceptable in the *NeanderThin* program, but people who find themselves unable to maintain fat loss may be eating too much sugar in the form of fruit. It is best to limit your intake of fruit until you reach your desired body composition, modeling your diet on that of hunter-gatherers to whom fruit is available only seasonally. Fruit as it occurs in nature is not as rich in sugar as the fruit bred and raised through agriculture. Don't make a meal of fruit. Treat it as dessert.

Artificial sweeteners. When any very sweet substance is consumed, the digestive and metabolic systems must be prepared before it reaches the stomach. The trigger mechanism for these changes is in the tongue. The taste of sweetness will slow the metabolic rate, alter the delicate balance of digestive enzymes and produce cravings--whether the sweetness comes from an artificial or a "natural" sweetener. Many artificial sweeteners have also been found to be carcinogenic and should be avoided for that reason alone.

Alcohol. Many people are thrown off the *NeanderThin* program by their inability to abstain from alcohol. Nachos and pizza seem almost inseparable from beer (the craving for each results from the same chemical reaction in the brain). And who drinks wine at cocktail parties without eating cheese? People who claim to be only social drinkers should remember that drinking tea or orange juice while everyone else has wine or beer or something stronger allows them to get more of what they socially drink for in the first place. Being alert while others are slightly inebriated or drunk leaves you in a better position to get a date or impress a potential client in the midst of your competitors.

Salt. As a hunter-gatherer, your taste for salt should diminish. Overconsumption of salt causes the body to retain water, thereby increasing blood pressure. On the *NeanderThin* diet your dietary sodium requirement will be easily satisfied through normal meat consumption.

Processed meats. Processed meats such as hot dogs, bacon, sausage and lunch meats are not forbidden. You should, however, avoid supermarket varieties which are prepared with sugar, corn syrup, salt and chemical preservatives. Besides being unhealthy these preservative technologies have become obsolete in the presence of modern refrigeration. If you cannot find a first-class butcher capable of making untainted varieties of these meats, make your own (which also happens to be far less expensive).

Eggs. Wild birds' eggs are the most preferable, free-range birds' eggs being the next most favorable, with factory-farm eggs being the least desirable. This is because the balance of amino acids and essential fatty acids is more favorable in the wild and free-range eggs. For this reason, people who have experienced egg allergies may find wild and free-range eggs to be more compatible with their digestion. People have debated whether fertile or infertile eggs are better. And while it is true that fertile eggs are actually healthier, the reason has nothing to do with the fertilization process. The difference is in what is fed to the mother. Eggs which are bred for fertility require a completely different and nutritionally superior food mixture in comparison to eggs which are bred for food production.

Coffee. In reality a burnt berry, coffee is popularly referred to as a bean because it is not edible raw and is, thus, forbidden on the *NeanderThin* program. To avoid the pangs of caffeine withdrawal substitute tea for coffee. The darker teas are higher in caffeine than green teas, but green teas are preferable as they are not fermented. Use caution with herbal teas as they have side effects. Try teas derived from mint or rose hips.

Wild game. Having lived in their natural habitats, wild animals are better sources of meat for humans than are domesticated animals, who are raised typically on grains and sometimes given injections of steroids and antibiotics. Meat from wild game is likely to be purer than meat from domesticated animals. All animals thrive on a natural diet. The animal that lives its entire life on a natural diet will to have a healthier body with a more beneficial lean to fat tissue composition, amino acids and enzymes. As well as being healthier, wild game tastes better and satisfies hunger longer than does commercial meat.

The act of hunting or fishing will also give you a more direct, spiritual connection to your food. By participating in the transformation of death into life which is the food chain, you will increase your participation in nature and have a greater interest in preserving wild places.

Wild plants. Hunting and gathering your own food provides a closer, more intimate relationship with your world. By foraging for berries, wild mushrooms, herbs, roots and other wild plants, you develop a closer connection to the natural world. You will see how the plants that are an important part of your diet have an even more important role as parts of a complex ecological system, and that as a human being you too have an environmental niche--that you are an integral, inseparable part of the natural world.

Hormonal imbalances. Women on birth control drugs or hormone replacement therapy during menopause may have problems losing body fat, as these therapies mimic pregnancy. They cause the body to retain fat. This effect may be overcome by physician-prescribed doses of the hormone testosterone or by the elimination of synthetic hormones altogether (the most natural solution).

Men taking female hormones or who have had one or both testicles removed for treatment of prostate or testicular cancer cannot pursue these options. The drawbacks of these therapies, however, can also be overcome by regular, strenuous exercise.

And finally,

NEVER CHEAT! Upon making the transition from a diet high in complex carbohydrates to one based on large amounts of animal protein and animal fat, "treating" yourself to a bag of potato chips, a bowl of ice cream or your favorite Mexican dish will have the opposite effect that it once did. What was once a satisfying meal or snack will probably make you sick. Carbohydrates have an addictive effect, and once you have given them up, indulging yourself will send you reeling. Because the immune system responds to even small doses, the smallest amounts of forbidden fruit may produce weight gains far out of proportion to their size. Some *NeanderThin* neophytes have reported gaining several pounds after eating only a single serving of rice or a small piece of cake. If you cannot stick to the diet religiously, you are better off not adopting it at all.

     If you do cheat, do not feel that all is lost and that you cannot continue the *NeanderThin* program. Depending on the amount and kind of forbidden fruit(s) consumed, there will be a period of time where you may feel uncomfortable if not very ill. This period of time should not last very long. Continue to pursue the *NeanderThin* program, and before long you will be back on track. An infrequent lapse in dietary vigilance can serve as excellent reinforcement for the devoted hunter-gatherer's commitment to his or her body and environment. This is not to say that any amount of cheating is encouraged or advised. Just remember that we are all human.

Resurrection
What To Expect

Any diet, no matter how natural, will require some adjustment, not only socially but also in the body's ability to process the new mix of nutrients being fed to it. A lifetime of eating unnatural foods has required the body to produce large amounts of digestive enzymes which a more natural diet would only require in small amounts. These enzymes are necessary to process large amounts of complex carbohydrates. The body must now learn to suppress these enzymes. The overproduction of these enzymes has also inhibited production of other enzymes and our bodies must now start producing these to process larger amounts of more natural foods such as meats and fats. As a result, large meals may produce a feeling of heaviness when this change is first undertaken. This will pass quickly as the body adjusts to a more natural balance.

When you change what goes in the body, what comes out changes as well. Bowel movements will change in both regularity and substance. Similar differences can been seen in the appearance of coyote scat and the feces left by domestic dogs fed commercial foods. Natural fecal matter has a looser consistency than that resulting from the incomplete digestion of unnatural foods. Natural foods are also processed faster and eliminated more quickly. The increase in frequency and looseness must not be mistaken for diarrhea. Soon the body will adjust and increased regularity will follow.

As the body learns to digest and eliminate natural foods more quickly, a strong increase in appetite will follow. This is often quite disconcerting to the new hunter-gatherer, although it is entirely natural and even desirable. This new hunger will make the new foods you are eating that much more satisfying. Preventing this hunger is easy--just eat! Hunger will slow the metabolism as it forces the body to put more energy into making fat, so it is to be avoided whenever possible. If it feels like you're eating all the time, you're well on your way to reaching your goals.

Do not mistake increased hunger for cravings. Cravings for forbidden foods are to be expected as all of these unnatural substances produce chemical addictions. These addictions are identical to the complex carbohydrate cravings of the alcoholic or heroin addict. Whether the source is a drug or a bagel, the endorphins (morphine-like substances) produced by the brain are the same, and it is these unnatural levels of endorphins which we crave. The feelings of fullness, well-being and tranquillity that are produced by these chemicals are most noticeable after a full agricultural feast such as Thanksgiving. You feel sleepy and lethargic--ready to watch football. In contrast, a large hunter-gather meal leaves you feeling energetic and ready to participate in a game of your own.

As with any addiction, withdrawal symptoms are to be expected. These may include nervousness, irritability, insomnia, irregular bowel movements and, most commonly, cravings for the forbidden substances. How cravings are dealt with will have a major impact on your ability to achieve the hunter-gather lifestyle.

The easiest way to eliminate cravings is to eliminate the offending substances completely. Just as the alcoholic must never take a drink, so must the hunter-gatherer eliminate even the smallest amount of forbidden fruit. If this is done religiously, cravings will soon subside completely. But even the smallest act of cheating will result in a high level of craving. Indeed, one potato chip will make you crave an entire bag (for about a week).

As cravings are stimulated by taste, even sugar substitutes such as aspartame or cyclamates may produce cravings of their own. Avoiding sugar-free foods completely will be far easier than trying to use them to wean yourself from sweets or sodas. Carbonated water is often a good substitute for those who crave sodas, but beware of unnaturally sweetened varieties masquerading as natural.

Cravings can be controlled through the use of high-fat snack foods. Eating pemmican, nuts, bacon or pork rinds (low-salt preferred) will greatly reduce the craving for sweets and provide an energy boost as well.

Maintaining this level of purity in your diet becomes easier with time as the body loses its unnatural cravings. The body will also increase its sensitivity to the forbidden fruits resulting in a feeling of illness if even the smallest amounts are eaten.

Given these cravings and increasing hunger, proper snacking is vital to maintaining the *NeanderThin* lifestyle. The best way to insure availability of proper snacks is to always carry a supply with you. Nuts, fruits and dried meats require no refrigeration and are easily carried in a pocket, purse or glove compartment. Carrying water is also a good idea as, often, only colas and beer are available at public events.

Eating between meals is to be encouraged, but it is also helpful to increase the size of each meal. People in general, but, especially former dieters, are hesitant at first to eat the increased portions required to satisfy *NeanderThin* needs. Some (especially women in our repressive society) may be embarrassed by the perception of others that they are overeating. Have faith that as your weight decreases, those looks of disapproval will change to looks of amazement.

It is important to remember to prepare meals with your new appetite in mind. Try to make more than you think you need. Having leftovers will provide a feeling of security as well as late-night snacks.

Of course, all of these adjustments will become easier as you see the results of the *NeanderThin* program. Any inconvenience will be offset by these results, and lifestyle changes will become second nature in a short time. For most people the benefits will be so great as to make any thought of returning to an agricultural diet unthinkable.

The most noticeable of these benefits, in most cases, is weight loss. This weight loss may be most dramatic in the initial adjustment period. Several pounds per week is not unusual. During this period it is very important to consume lots of water to forestall the effects of burning large amounts of body fats. This fat burning produces chemicals called ketones which are excreted in the breath and urine. By increasing liquid intake we make sure they come out through the urine and not the breath where they can produce an unpleasant odor.

Later, weight loss slows down and may even stall completely. Even a very small amount of cheating may produce such an episode. Should this occur, weight loss can be resumed by forcing the body to start producing ketones again. This can be accomplished by eliminating all carbohydrates (fruits and vegetables) completely. By becoming completely carnivorous for a period of 24-48 hours, the body will be forced to begin burning its stored fat. This process can be monitored by using urine test strips to detect the presence of ketones. Increased physical activity will also assist in accelerating weight loss.

It is not necessary to maintain the state of ketosis produced by an exclusive meat and fat diet.

As you reach a state of ketosis add small amounts of vegetable foods over the next few days until weight loss slows again and maintain that level. As your metabolism increases you may increase the vegetable portion again to taste.

Increasing physical activity is made easier by the increase in metabolic rate inherent in this program. This increase is due to the body having to spend less of its energy resources on immune responses to alien proteins in food. This energy is now available to be used in metabolic processes such as digestion, tissue regeneration and muscle development.

At first this new energy may feel somewhat uncomfortable. It may express itself as restlessness, nervousness, or insomnia. The solution is to increase your physical activity to match the increase in metabolic rate. As physical activity is increased, this discomfort will be eliminated. It will be replaced by the sense of calm and well-being associated with physical exertion, as opposed to the worn-out feeling associated with stress on the immune system.

The key to increasing physical activity is to make it convenient, interesting and habitual. Rather than spending twenty minutes driving to the gym, and changing your clothes once you arrive, it is far better to spend twenty minutes walking around the block. We are not talking about becoming an athlete, but rather getting yourself off the sofa. This should not be strenuous, sweaty exercise requiring a change of clothing. Take the time to meet your neighbors, walk the dog, improve your garden or watch birds. Interacting with your environment is a form of exercise in and of itself.

More important than any kind of exercise is changing one's personal habits and daily routine to include more physical activity. Walking up one flight of stairs several times a day is far better than thirty continuous minutes on a stair machine. Assign yourself parking based on your weight. Start at the furthest spot and move one space closer for every five pounds you lose. Get a dog that requires walking several times a day. Carry your own groceries to the car. Have more sex. Don't just sing in the shower-- dance too! Whatever you do, observe moderation. Keep in mind that the fastest-growing area of medicine is treating sports injuries. Pain is no gain, except for your doctor or masseur.

Any increase in energy will increase your appetite. With this in mind try to choose moderate physical activities that allow you to eat while you participate. Including a snack as part of your routine will make any activity more pleasurable and will extend the period of time that you devote to it.

As less of the body's energy is being consumed by immunological responses to alien proteins, more immunological resources are available to combat disease not attributable to dietary practices. In cultures that survive on technology-dependent foods exclusively (i.e., vegetarian cultures), diseases such as measles, mumps and influenza, which are considered minor in industrialized countries, result in extremely high mortality rates. In contrast, the hunter-gatherer experiences much milder colds, influenza, mononucleosis and yeast infections. Many people also notice that minor cuts and abrasions heal much faster.

Allergic reactions will also be reduced, but for a different reason. These particular immune reactions include itchy watery eyes, runny nose, asthma, sneezing, hives, dry skin, headaches, lethargy and swelling. All of these reactions are considered threshold phenomena; that is, until exposure to the allergen involved reaches a certain level, there is no response. But once that level is reached, the response is immediate and total. When one consumes alien proteins, the baseline is much closer to this threshold, resulting in allergic attacks to much smaller amounts of allergens than would affect a hunter-gatherer. From the evolutionary standpoint, it would be very difficult to survive a hay fever attack that affects your senses of sight, hearing and smell if you made your living as a hunter.

In conclusion, it should be noted that as dramatic as the results of *NeanderThin* are, the consequences of quitting are even more dramatic. Whether you decide to quit entirely or even partially, you will gain weight faster than ever before. The other health benefits which go along with the *NeanderThin* program will disappear as well.

Fortunately, if you have been following the program religiously, any amount of cheating will immediately result in illness. The nausea, lethargy, intestinal gas, constipation, fluid retention, etc. that will accompany an episode of cheating can serve as excellent reinforcement against cheating or quitting. If it feels bad, don't do it.

Book of Days
What I Ate Last Week

Monday

7:00 - Juice

2 Valencia oranges
1 tangelo
(juiced together in an inexpensive machine)

7:30 - Breakfast

8 strips bacon (uncured), fried
3 eggs over easy, fried in bacon grease

7:45 - Tea

1 cup English Breakfast tea
1 cup peppermint tea

10:30 - Snack

1 banana
1 cup lemon tea

12:00 - Lunch

2 baked chicken leg quarters (leftovers)
1 pear
1 glass unfiltered apple juice (available at most health food markets)

3:00 - Snack

1 ounce beef jerky
2 dates
1 cup generic tea

6:00 - Dinner

1 pound rib roast (smoked on grill)
1/4 pound of asparagus (steamed)
1 glass unfiltered apple juice

8:00
to
12:00 - Snack

1 quart nut mix (almonds, walnuts, pecans, dried apple bits, raisins, apricots, papaya)
3 glasses of carbonated water

Tuesday (on the road)

8:00 - Breakfast (roadside diner)	3 eggs scrambled 8 strips bacon (uncured) fried 1 cup tea 1 large orange juice
10:15 - Snack	1 ounce nut mix (see Monday) 1 apple 1 cup generic tea
12:00 - Lunch (barbecue restaurant)	1 pound barbecued ribs (no sauce) 2 orders cole slaw (very light mayonnaise) 1 glass iced tea
2:15 - Snack (7-11)	2 bananas 1 cup tea
7:00 - Dinner (restaurant)	1 16-ounce prime rib (cooked rare) tossed salad (no croutons, cheese, or dressing) 2 sliced apples 2 glasses Perrier
10:30 - Snack	1 pint nut mix 1 bottle Perrier

Wednesday (I go to the office.)

7:00 - Juice	1 grapefruit 1 tangelo (squeezed to juice)
7:45 - Breakfast	1 omelet (3 eggs, bacon (uncured), sausage, mushrooms, onions, tomatoes, green pepper) 2 cups green tea
10:30 - Snack (from briefcase)	3 slices summer sausage 1 pear
12:00 - Lunch (cafeteria)	baked fish (no breading) stewed spinach tossed salad (lettuce and tomatoes only) deviled egg fruit salad (drained) 2 glasses iced tea
3:00 - Snack (from briefcase)	dried fruit (pears, apples, banana chips) 1 cup generic tea
6:30 - Dinner	Cornish game hen (stuffed with mushrooms, celery, onion, chicken giblets, poultry seasoning) 2 carrots (raw) 1/2 cucumber (raw)
8:00 to 11:00 - Snack	nut mix 3 glasses carbonated water (flavored with juice of mandarin orange)

Thursday (I go hawking.)

7:00 - Juice	1 glass unfiltered pear juice
7:30 - Breakfast	3 pork chops (broiled) 1 banana
7:45 - Tea	2 cups English Breakfast tea
10:00 - Snack (from knapsack)	1 cup pemmican (dried venison meat, animal fat; see next section) 1 1/2 pint cider (hot in thermos)
12:30 - Lunch	1 small rabbit (caught by hawk, grilled on open fire) 1 fresh peach 1 fresh apple
3:30 - Snack (from knapsack)	1 cup pemmican 1 pear 1 cup green tea
7:00 - Dinner	1/2 roasted duck (stuffed with mushrooms, giblets, and onions) broccoli (steamed 5 minutes) 1 bowl unsweetened applesauce 2 cups hot cider
9:00 to 11:00 - Snack	leftover duck pieces several cups peppermint tea (w/ licorice root)

Friday (the big date)

8:30 - Juice	1 glass peach nectar (from health food store)
9:00 - Breakfast	1 12-ounce sirloin strip (cooked rare) 1/4 cantaloupe 1 cup raspberry tea
11:00 - Snack	1 kiwi 1 bag almonds
1:00 - Lunch (seafood restaurant)	1 dozen raw oysters 6 large shrimp tossed salad (lettuce, tomatoes, carrots, cucumber, radishes) 2 glasses iced tea
4:30 - Snack	handful sunflower seeds 1 plum 3 cups ginseng tea
7:00 - Dinner date (Mexican restaurant)	1 plate fajitas (no tortilla, no rice, no beans) 1 cup chili (no beans) 1/2 cup steamed carrots salad 2 glasses mineral water (French... it's a date!)
11:00 - Snack	fancy dried fruit (pears, peaches, cherries, two kinds of dates, figs) 2 cups peppermint tea several dollops peppermint oil applied directly on tongue

Saturday (the party)

9:00 - Juice   unfiltered grape juice

9: 30 - Breakfast   crab omelet (steamed crab claws for party)
Substitute crab meat for bacon and sausage in previous omelet.
1/8 honeydew melon
1/8 cantaloupe
1 small slice watermelon
Ball remaining melons for party.
2 cups green tea

11:00 - Snack   1 glass fresh-squeezed citrus juice (oranges, tangelos, grapefruit, limes)
Make additional citrus juice for party.

12:30 - Lunch   1 1/2 bowls chili (see recipe in next appendix)
Make enough for party as well.
bowl of strawberries
Clean remaining strawberries for party.

3:00 - Snack   nut mix (see previous recipe)
Make enough for party as well.
1 glass iced tea

5:00 - Snack   1/2 dozen smoked chicken wings
Make enough for party.
1 glass carbonated water
Chill the rest for party.

Party   Smoked beef brisket
smoked chicken wings
chili, steamed crab claws
fruit salad (melons, strawberries, bananas, cherries, apples, grapes)
citrus fruit punch (see midmorning snack, add carbonated water)
sliced raw veggies (celery, carrots, cucumber, broccoli, cauliflower, radishes, tomatoes)
NeanderThin guacamole (see next section)
nut mix, fancy dried fruit plate, pot of tea

Sunday (God and I kick back.)

10:30 - Juice	2 glasses citrus punch (Yes, it's even good flat.)
10:45 - Breakfast	1/2 dozen crab claws (party leftovers) bowl fruit salad 2 cups English Breakfast tea
1:00 - Lunch (light)	3 chicken wings 2 crab claws 1 small piece brisket raw veggie slices (All party leftovers)
3:00 to 5:30 - Football snack	nut mix citrus punch fruit salad dried fruit
7:00 - Dinner	beef brisket (served cold) tossed salad 1 small bowl chili 1 glass iced tea
10:00 - Snack	last of the brisket 1 glass iced herb tea

Food Rituals
Recipes

Chili

This legendary food, named "the state dish of Texas" by the Texas Legislature, has been a source of much debate, both as to the origin and the correct ingredients. It has been said by some of the most respected figures in the chili world that "anyone who would put beans in chili doesn't know beans about chili." Though probably more serendipitous than by design, chili is an ideal part of the *NeanderThin* diet. The following recipe is a "no frills" version. Included are a couple of the most common variations for the more adventurous who would "fly in the face" of Texas tradition.

Ingredients:
>   2 lbs. coarsely ground beef
>   2 oz. animal fat (beef suet or uncured bacon)
>   1/2 cup finely chopped onion
>   2 cloves garlic, minced
>   2 tablespoons chili powder (or more if desired)
>   1/2 teaspoon ground cumin (comino)
>   salt to taste
>   1/8 teaspoon dried oregano (optional)
>   water

1. In a large skillet (preferably cast-iron), render the fat over medium heat and remove the rinds.   Add

ground beef to skillet and cook until just brown. Add onion and garlic.

2. Add chili powder, cumin and oregano, and mix well. Add salt conservatively. (You can always add more water later if needed).

3. Reduce the heat to low and let simmer for at least 2 hours. The texture and flavor will change greatly as all of the ingredients blend together.

4. Add water as needed during cooking, keeping in mind that the final product should be somewhat thick.

Variation: Instead of adding water, add tomato juice or pureed tomatoes. Mushrooms and green peppers also make great additions.

A Vinegarless Vinaigrette

In the *NeanderThin* program, salads must be eaten without conventional condiments such as croutons, cheese and commercial salad dressings. Many people, however, find the idea of eating a "dry" salad unsavory. So the following is a recipe for a salad dressing that will add a great deal of flavor to any salad while remaining within the *NeanderThin* dietary guidelines.

Ingredients:
   1 clove garlic
   3 tablespoons olive oil
   1 tablespoon lemon juice
   1/2 teaspoon dry ground mustard

salt and freshly ground pepper to taste

1. Crush garlic clove and rub vigorously on the bottom of a small mixing bowl. Discard garlic. (If you are a big garlic fan, you may simply mince the clove and put it in the bowl.)
2. Add remaining ingredients to the bowl and whisk until all ingredients are thoroughly blended.

Note: This recipe is enough for 1 large or 2 small servings.

Waldorf Salad

This recipe will have a special place in the heart of any John Cleese/*Fawlty Towers* fan.

Ingredients:
  3 firm, crisp apples (red delicious, yellow
    delicious or a combination of the two)
  1 tablespoon of lemon juice (fresh-squeezed)
  1 cup celery, cut crosswise
  1/2 cup coarsely chopped walnuts
  1/2 cup homemade mayonnaise (see following
    recipe)
  1 1/2 tablespoon raw unfiltered honey
    (optional)
  lettuce leaves

1. Core and quarter apples and cut into 1/2" pieces. Put in a bowl and toss with lemon juice to coat. Add the celery and walnuts. Cover and chill.

2. Blend mayonnaise* and apple mixture together. If desired, serve on a bed of lettuce leaves.

* If using honey, blend with mayonnaise at this time.

Homemade Mayonnaise
(made in a blender or food processor)

Mayonnaise is a popular condiment and need not be abandoned by the modern hunter-gatherer. Commercially produced mayonnaise, however, is rife with chemicals and other undesirable ingredients and should be avoided for the most part. Homemade mayo, on the other hand, can be eaten without reservation, because all the ingredients used to make it are acceptable by *NeanderThin* standards.

Ingredients:
> 1 whole egg, at room temperature (plus 1 yolk
> for food processor)
> 1/2 teaspoon dry mustard
> 1/4 teaspoon salt (crushed sea salt is
> preferable)
> 1/4 teaspoon (preferably freshly ground) white
> pepper (optional)
> 1 1/2 tablespoons lemon juice (about 1 small
> lemon; 2 tablespoons for food
> processor)
> 1 cup light olive oil (plus 1/2 cup for food
> processor)

1. Break the eggs into the bowl of your blender or processor (use the steel blade). Add the dry mustard, salt, white pepper and lemon juice. Cover and blend 3 to 5 seconds.

2. With motor still running, remove the plastic stopper from the cover of the blender or the pusher from the food processor and begin adding the olive oil in a slow, steady stream until all of the oil is used. Blend only until mayonnaise is thick.

3. Scrape the mayonnaise into a glass container, cover and refrigerate (if the mayonnaise is not to be used up right away). The mayonnaise will keep for one week.

Spinach, Mushroom & Bacon Frittata

For those who like quiche, the Italian frittata is a wonderful substitute.

Ingredients:
>   1/2 lb. fresh raw spinach
>   1 lb. fresh mushrooms, sliced
>   1/3 cup olive oil
>   3-4 scallions, sliced thin
>   2 cloves garlic
>   1/2 teaspoon salt
>   1/2 teaspoon freshly ground black pepper
>   4-6 slices crisply cooked bacon (uncured),
>   crumbled
>   8 eggs, at room temperature

1. Carefully wash the spinach, and remove the stems. Place in a colander to drain. Slice the mushrooms thin.
2. In a 12" omelet pan, or a large skillet with sloping sides, heat 2 tablespoons of the olive oil over med-low heat. Add the scallions and the garlic and sauté until they have softened.
3. Add the sliced mushrooms, salt and pepper. Turn the heat to medium and sauté the mushrooms until they give up their liquid and it evaporates. Remove the pan from the heat to cool.
4. In a large mixing bowl, beat the eggs until they are light. Chop the drained spinach fine and add it to the eggs, then add the cooled mushroom mixture and the bacon. Stir to blend. Preheat the broiler.
5. Wipe the omelet clean with a paper towel and place it back on the stove over medium-high heat and add the olive oil. When the oil is hot, pour in the egg mixture. Quickly give the pan a few vigorous shakes back and forth across the burner surface to make sure the frittata does not stick; then immediately turn the meat to *very low* to avoid burning the bottom. Let cook for 20 minutes (more or less) *without* stirring.
6. When the egg mixture is set, but the top is still a little runny, remove the frittata from the stove and place it under the broiler for 1-2 minutes until the eggs have just set, but do not brown the top.
7. With the aid of a spatula, slide the frittata onto a serving platter and slice into wedges. The flavors of the vegetables will be more pronounced if you serve the frittata at room temperature.

Simple, Perfect Chicken Salad

A classic made *NeanderThin* style.

Ingredients:
>3 cups cooled cooked chicken removed from the bones and cut into bite-size pieces
>1 cup homemade mayonnaise (see earlier recipe)
>1 cup finely-chopped celery
>salad greens

Combine chicken, mayonnaise and celery in a large bowl and mix well. Serve on a bed of salad greens.

Optional garnishes:
1. Boiled eggs and parsley.
2. Walnut halves and watercress sprigs.
3. Almonds, green peppers and Italian parsley.

Tuna Salad with Onion, Avocado & Egg

Our tuna salad is made with gourmet-quality tuna packed in olive oil. Most commercial canned tuna is packed with either spring water or vegetable oil and contains an ingredient called hydrolyzed vegetable protein, which is often derived from corn. Such low-grade canned tunas should be avoided. If you are unable to find tuna which is not packed in unacceptable methods and does not contain forbidden substances, try substituting fresh tuna or even chicken in this recipe instead.

Ingredients:

> 1 head lettuce; washed, dried and separated into leaves
> 2 7 oz. cans imported Italian tuna, packed in olive oil *
> 1 cup onion rings
> 1 cup diced avocado
> 4 hard-boiled eggs, quartered
> 2-3 tablespoons capers (optional)
> 1/2 to 3/4 cup vinegarless vinaigrette (refer to earlier recipe)

Put the greens in a large salad bowl, and place the tuna, onions, avocados and eggs on top. Dress with the vinaigrette.

* If imported tuna is unavailable, substitute 14 oz. fresh tuna or chicken. Add approximately 1/2 cup of olive oil and toss.

NeanderThin Guacamole

Use guacamole as a dip for other snack foods or as a dressing or condiment.

Ingredients:

> 4 large ripe avocados
> 4 tablespoons fresh-squeezed lemon juice

1 cup minced onion
1 cup chopped fresh tomato
4 sprigs fresh cilantro or parsley
4 small hot chili peppers, minced
4 teaspoons minced garlic
salt to taste

Slice the avocados lengthwise, remove the pits, and scrape the fruit into a bowl. Mash the fruit with a fork, add the remaining ingredients, and blend thoroughly. This recipe makes 4 cups.

Deviled Eggs

Ray's secret weapon.

Ingredients:
8 hard-boiled eggs
3 tablespoons mayonnaise (see earlier recipe)
1/4 teaspoon dry mustard
6 slices bacon (uncured), fried and crumbled
Salt to taste

1. Slice eggs lengthwise. Separate yolks and whites, placing yolks in a bowl.
2. Combine mayonnaise, mustard, bacon and salt with yolks. Blend until the mixture takes on a smooth consistency.
3. Spoon mixture into egg whites. Cover and chill if eggs are not meant to be eaten immediately.

Chicken Soup

Nothing is more filling or warming on a cold winter morning than a bowl of chicken soup.

Ingredients:
> 1 whole chicken with giblets
> 4 stalks celery
> 2 large carrots
> 1 onion
> 1/2 teaspoon poultry seasoning

In a large pot add deboned chicken, giblets, chopped vegetables and poultry seasoning. Add enough water to cover everything. Bring to a boil. Then let simmer for 15 minutes. Serve hot.

Beef Soup

Favored by Arctic explorers for ease of preparation and as a source of energy and warmth.

Ingredients:
> 1 cup water
> 2 tablespoons hamburger
> (or 1 tablespoon of pemmican)

Bring water to a boil. Stir in hamburger or pemmican until water boils again. Serve.

Cornish Game Hen

One of Ray's favorites.

Ingredients:
>1 whole chicken with giblets
>4 stalks celery
>1 cup fresh mushrooms
>1/4 cup *real* bacon (uncured) bits
>1/2 onion
>1 teaspoon poultry seasoning
>4 tablespoons bacon (uncured) grease

1. Wash chicken and stuff with seasoned, chopped giblets and vegetables.
2. Smear seasoned bacon grease on outside of chicken and place in roasting pan.
3. Bake at 350 degrees for 20 minutes per pound of chicken plus 20 minutes for stuffing.
4. Baste every 30 minutes to taste.

Beef Jerky

Jerked meat makes a convenient snack food for road trips or carrying to the office, and it is quite simple to make.

Ingredients:
As much red meat (beef, venison) as you want.

Classically, jerky is made by removing all fat from the meat, cutting meat into 1/4" strips and

101

laying the strips out to dry in the sun for 1 to 2 days. If you elect to use an oven, heat (do not cook) the strips at a very low temperature until they are thoroughly dried. (A food dehydrator is preferable.)

As *NeanderThin* jerky is not sugar-cured and contains no preservatives, it may become moldy in a warm, humid environment. If you want to keep it for an extended period of time (more than a week), store it in your freezer.

Pemmican

Pemmican was relied on heavily by native North Americans when traveling. A high energy food which keeps for an extended period of time, pemmican also makes a great snack for the urban hunter-gatherer.

Ingredients:
> 1 lb. suet (beef fat)
> 1 lb. dried red meat (lean uncooked; remove all fat before drying; 6 lbs. raw lean meat yields 1 lb. dried meat)

1. Render (melt) the suet in a (preferably cast-iron) pan. The suet must be rendered twice to prevent spoilage.
2. Pound dried meat into a fine powder (a food processor can make this process much easier) and add to the rendered suet.

102

3. While the mixture is still liquid, pour into muffin pan to make pemmican cakes.

Additional Tips:
1. Wrap cakes in wax paper for convenience, as pemmican is greasy.
2. Dried berries can be added for taste.

Mom's Catsup

The *NeanderThin* approved version of America's favorite vegetable. (Submitted by Ray's mom who, although in her seventies, is a *NeanderThin* convert and is not to be trifled with!)

Ingredients:
> 3 1/3 lbs. tomatoes (washed and sliced)
> 2 medium sized sliced onions
> 1/8 clove garlic
> approximately 1/2 bay leaf (small)
> 1/2 red pepper

Boil these ingredients until they are soft. Strain them, and add:
> 1/4 cup unsweetend juice (select the naturally
> sweeter ones: white grape, pear, or
> apple)

In a spice bag add the following:
> 1 teaspoon whole allspice (scant)
> 1 teaspoon whole cloves
> 1 teaspoon whole mace

> 1 teaspoon celery seed
> 1 teaspoon black peppercorns
> 1/2 inch stick cinnamon

The spices may be varied. Add spice bag to mixture, boiling the ingredients quickly, stirring frequently until they are reduced to 1/2 the quantity. Remove spice bag.

Add:

> 1/2 cup lemon juice (fresh squeezed)
> cayenne and course salt if desired

Boil the catsup for 10 more minutes. Bottle* catsup at once in clean jars leaving 1/2 to 3/4 inch of headroom.** Cover and freeze immediately. Always refrigerate container of catsup that is in use.

*Choose containers (plastic or glass) of a size that your family will use in a week's time. Since there are no preservatives added, the catsup can spoil.

**Headroom allows for freezer swell.

NeanderThin Barbecue Sauce

The crown jewel of the *NeanderThin* kitchen.

Ingredients:

> 2 tablespoons bacon fat
> 2 cloves garlic, minced
> 2 tablespoons onions, finely chopped

1 teaspoon chili powder (or more, to taste)
1 can tomato paste
1/2 cup water
6 oz. apple juice concentrate (100% natural)
1 teaspoon dried rosemary leaves, crushed
1/2 teaspoon coriander seeds, finely ground
        or crushed
1 teaspoon ground ginger
juice from 1 orange, 1/3-1/2 cup (more or less)

1. Sauté garlic and onion in bacon fat over med-low heat until tender (5-10 minutes).
2. Add chili powder, rosemary, coriander and ginger.
3. Add all other ingredients and stir until well blended.
4. Simmer over low heat for at least 30 minutes to let flavors blend. If sauce becomes too thick, add water.

Baked Chicken with Herbs

Ingredients:
        one 3-4 lb. chicken
        2 tbs.. olive oil
        salt and pepper to taste (both optional)
        2-3 tsp.. dried herb of your choice
                (rosemary, thyme, tarragon, sage, etc.)

1. Preheat oven to 350 degrees.
2. Wash chicken and pat dry with paper towels.
3. Rub skin of chicken with olive oil. (If using salt or pepper or both, coat chicken evenly with them now.)

4. To bring out the flavor of the dried herb (use only one at a time), rub vigorously back and forth in palms or crush in a mortar.

5. Rub entire surface of chicken with herb.

6. Place in baking dish large enough to hold, breast side up.

7. Bake at 350 degrees for approximately 1 1/2 hours total. After first 1/2 hour check for juices in pan. Once juices appear baste chicken about every 15-20 minutes until done. Chicken is done when meat thermometer placed in the thickest part of the meat (not touching a bone) reads 185 degrees, or when leg joint doesn't wiggle and juices from pierced leg-thigh joint are clear (the best way to learn how to tell when a chicken is done is to cook a few and learn). If you doubt your ability, investing in a $3 meat thermometer will save you much time and guessing.

Variation: If you want to give the chicken more flavor, mix the juice of one lemon with the olive oil, and put the two halves of the lemon rind in the chicken's cavity during the baking (remove rind before serving).

Venecian Salad

This is a well-balanced salad, sure to please lovers of Italian food.

Ingredients:
    1 head Romaine lettuce, bruised outer
        leaves removed

1 bunch arugula, stems trimmed
1 green pepper, julienned
1 tomato, cut into wedges
6 mushrooms, sliced thin
1/2 cucumber, sliced thin
1/2 bunch seedless grapes, halved
1/4 cup extra virgin olive oil
juice of 1/2 lemon
salt and freshly ground black pepper to taste

Combine the vegetables and grapes in a large salad bowl. Add the olive oil and lemon juice. Add salt and pepper to taste. Toss gently.

Pesto

Pesto is a delicious fresh Italian pasta sauce, but it makes an equally good sauce for chicken or fish or a dip for vegetables. It will store almost indefinitely in the refrigerator if you put it in a container and pour a little olive oil on top of it.

Ingredients:
6 tablespoons good quality extra virgin
    olive oil
1 cup shelled walnuts (or if you want a
    richer sauce, replace up to 1/2 of
    the walnuts with pine nuts)
4 cups tightly-packed fresh basil
3 tablespoons Italian parsley
salt and freshly-ground black pepper to taste

Place all ingredients in a blender or food processor and blend until just combined.

Pesto can also be used to flavor chicken or fish that is baked or grilled. Simply brush a light coat of pesto on the meat and cook as usual.

Try adding pesto to any broth-based soup (such as the "Roman Egg Drop Soup" recipe herein). Just add a tablespoon or so at a time until it suits you.

Lemon Thyme Pesto Chicken

Ingredients:
> one 3-4 lb. chicken
> 2 tablespoons thyme (dried or ,if available,
>   6 tablespoons fresh)
> juice of 1/2 small lemon
> 2-3 tablespoons extra virgin olive oil
> salt and freshly-ground black pepper to taste
> 1 clove garlic, minced

1. Preheat oven to 350 degrees.
2. Combine all ingredients (except chicken) and mix thoroughly. (The best way is to grind them is with a mortar and pestle, but if you don't have one, put everything in a small bowl and stir vigorously so as to release the essential oils from the thyme and garlic.)
3. Coat chicken with mixture and bake at 350 degrees for approximately 1 1/2 to 2 hours. After the first hour the chicken should begin to release its

juices. Baste the chicken with the juices every 15 to 20 minutes until done.

If you have already prepared pesto (see previous recipe), you can coat the chicken with it and cook the chicken in the manner described above.

Pork Chops Mexican Style

Ingredients:
>   4 pork chops (1 to 1 1/2 inches)
>   4 tablespoons bacon fat
>   1 medium onion, chopped
>   2 cloves garlic, finely chopped
>   1 teaspoon ground cumin
>   1 teaspoon oregano
>   1 1/2 teaspoons salt
>   1 cup tomato sauce
>   2 tablespoons chili powder

Heat fat in large skillet over medium heat. When grease is hot, brown pork chops. When chops are brown, add onion and garlic, and sauté until soft. Add oregano, cumin and salt. Add tomato sauce, cover, and allow to simmer for 10 minutes. Uncover, add chili powder, and turn chops. Simmer 10 more minutes or until tender.

Roman Egg Drop Soup

Ingredients:
    4 cups chicken broth
    2 cups chopped and washed fresh spinach
    2 eggs, beaten
    1 tablespoon grated lemon rind
    salt and pepper to taste

Bring broth to a boil, add spinach, and boil gently for several minutes. Mix eggs, lemon rind, salt and pepper. Lower heat, stir in eggs, and cook for a minute or so while the eggs set. Serves three.

Catechism
Frequently Asked Questions

Q: Should I consult my physician before starting *NeanderThin*?

A: *It will not hurt to get a good summary of your current health status in order to chart any improvements.   As your body cannot require anything that, in nature, it cannot acquire, your doctor should have no problem with* NeanderThin, *no matter what your condition.*

Those wishing to begin the NeanderThin *program under medical supervision should contact:*
Dr. Michael R. Eades
Arkansas Center for Health and Weight Control
11025 Anderson Drive, Ste. 130
Little Rock, Arkansas 72212
Dr. Eades has done extensive research on Paleolithic Nutrition and has many years in counseling weight loss patients.   He may also be able to recommend a physician in your area familiar with Paleolithic Nutrition.

Q: Don't the high levels of red meat and animal fats in the *NeanderThin* program lead to cardiovascular disease?

A: *Although* NeanderThin *seems high in fat at first glance, by removing vegetable oils (corn, soybean, peanut, canola, etc.), trans-fatty acids (hydrogenated vegetable oils such as margarine), and dairy fats (milk, butter, heavy cream), it turns out to be equal to or lower in fat than the average American diet.   Approximately half the fat in red*

111

meat consists of stearic acid, a powerful antioxidant, which reduces your risk of both arteriosclerosis and cancer. Remember that heart disease is an immune system problem caused by the ingestion of alien proteins, not saturated fat.

Practicing NeanderThin has been shown to improve blood cholesterol ratios (LDL/HDL and Total Cholesterol/HDL). For a complete explanation of how this works see Protein Power, the book by Drs. Michael and Mary Dan Eades (as referenced in the bibliography). Chapter 7, "Cholesterol Madness," of the Eades' book shows why eating red meat will not clog your arteries.

Trying to reduce fat consumption while following the principles of the NeanderThin program will only reduce metabolism, produce fatigue and slow weight loss. Low-fat diets have been shown to dramatically increase LDL ("bad") cholesterol and lipid levels in some individuals (see Garg/JAMA article referenced in bibliography). Remember that fat from natural sources is not the culprit--it is the immune system's response to unnatural foods that causes autoimmune disease (such as heart disease).

Q: I'm not overweight. Why should I eat this way?
A: Most people who adopt NeanderThin are not overweight (at least for very long). Even a person of average weight will experience dramatic improvements in their overall health, energy level and fitness within a few weeks of adopting the NeanderThin program.

Even if you are not presently overweight your genetics may betray you twenty years from now. By eating like a hunter-gatherer you greatly reduce your *risk of succumbing to autoimmune disease (95% of Americans die of autoimmune diseases).*

You will not become too thin eating this way. Once you have reached your optimal body composition, you will remain there as long as you follow the program.

The NeanderThin *view also provides environmental, spiritual and political benefits for many.*

Q: To lose weight should I reduce my fat intake?
A: *No. If you are trying to lose weight you are trying to metabolize your own body fats. As your own fat is an animal fat, it is important to trigger this metabolic process by ingesting animal fat.*

Q: As *NeanderThin* cuts out whole categories of food, should I take vitamin and mineral supplements?
A: *Vitamins are enzymes used by the body to metabolize food. When you eat unnatural foods they are used up faster than the body can replace them. This leads to vitamin deficiencies. By avoiding the forbidden fruits and eating a wide variety of natural foods, the need for vitamin and mineral supplements is eliminated.*

Q: *NeanderThin* seems awfully strict. Aren't there easier ways to lose weight?
A: *The only other way to lose weight involves caloric restriction and regular strenuous exercise. Like* NeanderThin, *this regimen must be continued for a lifetime to keep the weight off. The resulting hunger from starvation rations and the high risk of injury*

if not impossible for most who try it. With NeanderThin *the cravings for forbidden fruits diminish with time, but with caloric restriction you will always be hungry and will never be allowed to eat your fill. Also, the high injury rates associated with exercise programs have made sports medicine the fastest growing medical specialty.*

Q: My dog is overweight. Will *NeanderThin* work for him?

A: *In nature wolves and humans eat essentially the same things. (In fact, some scientists postulate this as the reason for wolves becoming the first domesticated animals.)* NeanderThin *table scraps supplemented by raw meat (I use beef heart) will provide the optimum diet for your dog and have him in good shape very soon.*

Q: Can I still drink alcohol?

A: *All alcohol (yeast urine) is forbidden fruit and must be avoided. Ingesting herbs is the preferred method of intoxication for hunter-gatherers everywhere in the world.*

Q: Is *NeanderThin* safe during pregnancy?

A: *As hunter-gatherers have the easiest births and the lowest incidence of birth defects, it is not only safe but is preferred.*

The pregnant woman craves added nutrients to nourish and sustain herself and her developing baby. The mother's immune system is also working hard to protect mother and child, so care must be taken to avoid the forbidden fruits while satisfying cravings by increasing dietary diversity. In this way the nausea common in pregnancy can be greatly reduced if not eliminated. And by increasing her intake of acceptable plant foods (fruits, veggies and nuts) the mother will avoid ketosis.

Q: Since the inception of technology, hasn't the human body evolved to allow consumption of the forbidden fruits?

A: *Technology-dependent foods have been eaten by mankind for less than 10,000 years. This amount of time equals approximately 300 generations. There are several breeds of chickens available with much longer pedigrees than humans, all of which thrive on essentially the same blend of nutrients optimal for their jungle forbears.*

Even small evolutionary changes take hundreds of thousands of years (some scientists say millions of years) to occur. For humans to adapt to foods that are not edible to any other primate would involve vast changes in our immune system as expressed in our DNA. To mutate to a form outside one's own order (Primata) would be considered a huge evolutionary change. We are essentially the same creatures we were before the Neolithic Revolution.

Q: How long will it take me to lose weight using *NeanderThin*?

A: *It depends upon how overweight you are and how long it took you to become that way. If you are very heavy initial weight loss may be very dramatic (3-5 pounds per week). As you approach your ideal weight, this loss will slow and the last 10 or 20 pounds may take much longer (2-3 years). The process may be accelerated by lowering intake of high-carbohydrate foods (dried fruits, juices, nuts) and increasing moderate exercise (walking, golf, avoiding elevators, power parking, etc.). Adding muscle mass to your body through strength training will also increase your metabolism and speed weight loss.*

Q: I love animals. Can I practice *NeanderThin* as a vegetarian?
A: *No. Without red meat the human body lacks the enzymes to process iron. Iron deficiency is responsible for the high incidence of retardation, birth defects and weakened physical condition endemic in vegetarian societies. Without the proteins contained in the forbidden fruits (grains, beans, dairy products), severe protein deficiencies will occur which could be life-threatening.*

As the principle cause of animal extinction and death is the plow and not the slaughterhouse, vegetarians actually kill more animals through starvation and habitat destruction than does the meat-eater through his dietary habits. In fact, it is for this reason that the person wearing a fur coat has killed less than 10% of the animals killed by person wearing a cotton coat (cotton is one of the most ecologically damaging crops grown today, second only, perhaps, to rice.). Perhaps the only species that are not endangered in our modern world are the domestic animals we eat.

116

Q: Once I have reached my weight goal, can I return to normal foods?

A: *No. Any weight lost will be regained even more quickly than it was originally lost. It cannot be overemphasized that it is not the calories or fat content that produces the weight gain, as has been traditionally proposed; instead, it is the alien proteins present in the forbidden fruits which causes an overweight condition.*

Q: According to your theory, shouldn't I eat all my food raw?

A: *In a perfect world, yes. But modern farming and food processing techniques preclude this practice. Meats, poultry, eggs and seafood are prone to contamination by bacteria (salmonella, e. coli, etc.) and parasites (trichinosis, tapeworms, etc.) and should be cooked or dried at least enough to sterilize them. When available, irradiated foods will eliminate this risk and make steak tartar and raw eggs much more popular. The slight loss of vitamins and nutrients caused by light cooking can be compensated for by fruit and vegetables in the diet, but these should be washed thoroughly to remove bacteria, germs and pesticide residue.*

Q: Are prepackaged convenience foods (frozen, canned, microwaveable, etc.) allowed in the *NeanderThin* program?

A: *Although not categorically eliminated, most prepackaged foods contain one or more of the forbidden fruits and should be avoided. On a case by case basis, this can only be determined by carefully reading labels. Because of their low government subsidy costs, unnatural foods are often used as cheap fillers in a wide variety of products. Often, soy is added to meat products, flavored corn syrup is substituted in fruit juices and starch from corn is added to almost anything.*

Some prepackaged foods such as frozen fruit juices are lacking for what is not there. Fruit juice from concentrate has had most of the fiber, protein and vitamins removed, leaving only the sugar and should, therefore, not be seen as a substitute for real fruit juice or fresh fruit.

Q: I have food allergies. Will this diet work for me?
A: *As the most common food allergies are reactions to corn, wheat and milk, NeanderThin should be excellent for individuals suffering from conditions caused by their consumption. Less common are allergic reactions to seafood. As these were among the last foodstuffs added to the human diet, this is not unexpected. Should you have these allergic reactions, seafood must still be avoided.*

Individuals who experience allergies to other foods such as eggs, certain nuts and fruits should continue to avoid these foods. Fear not, however, as, regardless of the severity of the food allergy, acceptable substitutes can always be found and the NeanderThin program continued.

Q: Won't my friends think that I'm weird if I eat this way?
A: *At first, yes, as you are going against thousands of years of cultural programming; but as your condition improves, any disdain will replaced by curiosity. As your condition improves, you will also*

become more prone to zealotry, which fat people may find obnoxious. Try to avoid this by not criticizing everything they eat. Instead, lead by example.

Q: Isn't *NeanderThin* expensive?
A: *It may seem that way at first. For the price of a pound of meat, one can buy a bushel of government-subsidized wheat. But by eating out less and avoiding unnecessary medical costs associated with the forbidden fruits, the hunter-gatherer comes out ahead. Remember that slim people get more raises and make more money, and people with disabilities caused by immune system diseases often make no money at all. There is no better investment than your own body.*

Q: Shouldn't I exercise more?
A: *Yes, but only in moderation. Strenuous exercise has more risks than benefits and should be avoided. The best exercise is walking, bearing in mind that it is the time spent and not the distance covered that counts. Any activity pursued with this rule of thumb in mind--such as dog walking, bird watching, falconry, golf, etc.--is excellent.*

Mental activity is also a form of exercise. Try to use your increased energy to improve and not just entertain--i.e., distract--your mind. This will improve not only your physical health but may also improve your intellectual abilities and overall outlook on life.

Q: Is *NeanderThin* good for children?
A: *As many childhood conditions such as obesity, hyperactivity, ear infections, frequent colds, juvenile diabetes, juvenile epilepsy, rickets, myopia, etc. have been shown to be diet-related,* NeanderThin *is excellent for children. For the same reasons, breast feeding is also highly recommended.*

Children are often tempted by such goodies as milk and cookies served by well-meaning day care workers, teachers or friends' parents. They must be educated from a very early age to avoid the forbidden fruits at all costs.

Q: Why have I not heard of this before?
A: *Quite simply, it is a question of perspective. As modern humans, we tend to view all things through the lens of civilization. Our worldview is framed by a certain set of social and cultural parameters of which we are largely unaware and which distort our understanding of our biological and evolutionary origins.*

What we call civilization is a continuous process, the origins of which lie in agrarian agricultural intensification. Cultures founded upon agrarian agricultural intensification began in several parts of the world, including the Fertile Crescent of the Middle East, the Indus River Valley of India, the Yellow River Valley of China, the valley of Mexico and the high plateaus of Peru.

Just as the Roman Empire was built for the production and distribution of bread and wine, so all civilizations promote activities that benefit the crop species that spawn them. The peculiarities of the life cycles of different crops are often used by anthropologists to explain the differences found between cultures.

Agricultural plant species promote themselves through custom, religion, politics, manners, morals and ethics. Since Gutenberg they have also used the mass media. Indeed a large part of all advertising is paid for by the forbidden fruits.

Hunter-gatherers and their views do not fit into agrarian civilizations very well. Perceived as threatening, they are the untouchables, the unclean, the heathens. They have suffered genocide and slavery when they have come in contact with civilized man.

The hunter-gatherer viewpoint is often contrary to cultural norms. Such events as corporate dinners and certain religious ceremonies require great tact if forbidden fruit is to be refused without offense.

When you tell your doctor "It hurts when I eat forbidden fruit," he is unlikely to say, "So don't eat forbidden fruit." He is going to try to find a medicine that will allow you to eat a favorite food. After all, medicine is the name of the game, and your doctor does not want you to miss any of the benefits of civilization.

Vegetarians and animal rights activists will try to convince you that land now devoted to cattle (which also supports wild animals, birds, insects and other crop eaters) should be planted fence to fence with beans or grain.

Just as the English House of Lords favored the large agrarian landholder, so the Great Compromise of 1787 has insured that the U. S. Senate gives greater representation to farmers than to urban tenants and building owners. This unequal balance of power only increases as the number of farmers becomes smaller in relationship to city populations (farmers presently make up approximately 1% of the population of the U. S.).

Also, the government promotes a food pyramid, favoring the forbidden fruits, which was brought about by the same sort of political forces that built the original pyramids.

All of the aforementioned forces have served to overwhelm the quiet voice of NeanderThin *Man, leaving his views underrepresented in ethnic and anthropological studies. The chief reason, however, that you might not have heard of the Paleolithic diet before may simply be that in our modern, high-tech world, the simplest ideas and solutions often lie hidden in plain sight.*

It is only since civilization has begun to face worldwide ecological disaster, caused by agricultural intensification, that the hunter-gatherer viewpoint has come to light, finding its voice in both the Deep Ecology movement and the new science of Paleolithic Nutrition.

Q: Is *NeanderThin* good for the environment?
A: *Since ancient times, the most destructive factor in the degradation of the environment has been monoculture agriculture. The production of wheat in ancient Sumeria transformed once-fertile plains into salt flats that remain sterile 5000 years later. As well as depleting both the soil and water sources, monoculture agriculture also produces environmental damage by altering the delicate balance of natural ecosystems. World rice*

production in 1993, for instance, caused 155 million cases of malaria by providing breeding grounds for mosquitoes in the paddies. Human contact with ducks in the same rice paddies resulted in 500 million cases of influenza.

Many environmentalists now believe the only way to preserve the environment is to return to our natural place on the food chain (tree of life). Over time nature produces more nutrients per acre than any method of agriculture. Learning to intelligently harvest this natural bounty without destroying it is the biggest challenge facing modern man.

Bibliography
As It Is Written

Only through hunting and gathering knowledge will your path lead you to the meaning of life.

ARTICLES

Aiello, Leslie C. and Peter Wheeler, "The Expensive Tissue Hypothesis: The Brain and the Digestive System in Human and Primate Evolution." *Current Anthropology* vol. 36, #2 (April 1995) 199-221.
(Analyzes human gut morphology and how eating meat made us smart .)

Ames, B.N., "Ranking Possible Carcinogenic Hazards" *Science* 236 (April 17, 1987) 271-80.

Ames, B.N., "Paleolithic Diet, Evolution and Carcinogens", *Science* 238 (Dec. 18, 1987) 1633-34.

Ames, B.N., "Carcinogenic Risk Estimation" *Science* 240 (May 20, 1988) 1043-47.
(Series of articles by one of the leading authorities on the causes of cancer. Ames shows how common foods may pose a greater threat of cancer than some of the chemicals often labeled carcinogenic.)

Atkinson, Mark A., Noel K. Maclaren, "What Causes Diabetes?" *Scientific American* (July 1990) 62-71.

Bishop, Jerry E., "More Fatty Foods Are Backed in Test of Diabetic Diets." *Wall Street Journal* (May 11, 1994).

Boehmer, Harald von, Pawel Kisielow, "How the Immune System Learns about Self." *Scientific American* (Oct. 1991) 74-81.

Bower, B., "The 2-million-year-old meat and marrow diet resurfaces." *Science News* (Jan. 3, 1987) 7.

Bryant, Vaughn, "I Put Myself on a Caveman Diet-Permanently." *Prevention* Vol. 31 No. 9 (1979) 128-137.

_____, "Eating Right Is an Ancient Rite." *Natural Science* (Jan. 1995) 216-221.

_____, "Prehistoric Diets." *University Lecture Series, Texas A &M University* (Nov. 28, 1979).

_____, "The Paleolithic Health Club." *1995 Yearbook of Science and the Future* (1994) published by Encyclopedia Britannica, Inc., Chicago. 114-133.
(Vaughn Bryant is the head of the Department of Anthropology at Texas A & M University and is also a professor of biochemistry.)

Cerami, Anthony, Helen Vlassara and Michael Brownlee, "Glucose and Aging." *Scientific American* (May 1987) 90-96.

Centofanti, M., "Diabetes complications: More than sugar?" *Science News* Vol. 148 (Dec. 23 & 30, 1995) 421.

Cohen, Leonard A., "Diet and Cancer." *Scientific American* (Nov. 1987) 42-48.

Diamond, Jared, "THE WORST MISTAKE IN THE HISTORY OF THE HUMAN RACE." *Discover* (May 1987) 64-66.
(Explains how the invention of agriculture caused war, disease, oppression and the income tax..)

Diamond, Jared, "THE GREAT LEAP FORWARD." *Discover* (May 1989) 50-60.
(Describes the Neolithic Revolution.)

Dolnick, Edward, "Beyond the French paradox." *Health* (October 1992) 40.
(Explains how the French have a high-fat diet and have very little heart disease.)

Dunbar, Robin, "Foraging for nature's balanced diet; finding the link between diet and longevity among human and animal groups." *Focus* (Aug. 31, 1991) 25-?

Eaton, S. B., Melvin Konner, "PALEOLITHIC NUTRITION: A Consideration of Its Nature and Current Implications." *The New England Journal of Medicine* Vol. 312 No. 5 (Jan. 31, 1985) 283-289.
(MUST READ!!!)

Frisch, Rose E., "Fatness and Fertility." *Scientific American* (March 1988) 88-95.

Garg, Abhimanyu, M.B.B.S., M.D. *et al*, "Effects of Varying Carbohydrate Content of Diet in Patients With Non-Insulin-Dependent Diabetes Mellitus." *Journal of the American Medical Association* vol. 271, #18 (May 11, 1994) 1421-1428.
(Shows how a low-carbohydrate diet caused a rapid increase in LDL-cholesterol levels in insulin-resistant--i.e., overweight--patients.)

Henry, Linda, "Wild Side: Bodybuilders advance to primitive protein for lean muscularity." *Muscle & Fitness* (March 1994) 85...

Hopkins, Susan, "Eating the caveman's high-fiber diet can be healthy." *The Battalion* Vol. 74 No. 179 (Thursday, July 23, 1981) 1.

Johnson, Mary Ann, "The Georgia Centenarian Study: Nutritional Patterns of Centenarians." *The International Journal of Aging & Human Development* Vol. 34(1) (1992) 57-76.
(Explains that hundred-year-olds typically eat high-fat diets.)

Krajick, Kevin, "Waiter, There's a Fly in My Soup, and I Ordered the Cricket Salad." *Newsweek* (Sept. 20, 1993) 59E.

Larkin, Marilynn, "CAVE CUISINE." *Health* (Nov. 1985) 37-38.

Leonard, Wm. R., Marcia L. Robertson, "Evolutionary Perspectives on Human Nutrition: The Influence of Brain and Body Size on Diet and Metabolism." *American Journal of Human Biology* Vol. 6 (1994) 77-88.
(Similar to Aiello's "Expensive Tissue Hypothesis...")

Lieb, Clarence W., M.D., "The Effects on Human Beings of a Twelve Months' Exclusive Meat Diet." *Journal of the American Medical Association* (July 6, 1929) 20-22.
(Stefansson's famous year-long experiment with an all-meat diet at Bellview Hospital in New York.)

Lowenstein, Jerold M., "Who ate what when." *Oceans* (June 1988) 72.

McKie, Robin, "Meaty evidence: Steak made humans smart." (quotes *Current Anthropology* journal) *London Observer Service* (Jan. 14, 1995).

Mead, Nathaniel, "Don't Drink Your Milk!" *Natural Health* (July/August 1994) 70-73, 112.

Milton, Katharine, "Diet and Primate Evolution." *Scientific American* (August 1993) 86-93.

Molleson, Theya, "The Eloquent Bones of Abu Hureyra." *Scientific American* (Aug. 1994) 70-75.

O'Dea, Kerin, Ph.D. *et al*, "Impaired Glucose Tolerance, Hyperinsulinemia and Hypertriglyceridemia in Australian Aborigines from the Desert." *Diabetes Care* Vol. 11, No. 1 (Jan. 1988) pp. 23-29.
(Compares effects of urban life and hunter-gathering on Australian Aborigines.)

Raloff, J., "Obesity, diet linked to deadly cancers." *Science News* Vol. 147 No. 3 (Jan. 21, 1995) 39.

_____ "High-fat diets help athletes perform." *Science News* Vol. 149 (May 4, 1996) 287.

Rennie, John, "THE BODY AGAINST ITSELF." *Scientific American* (Dec. 1990) 107-15.

Richardson, Sarah, "MEDICINE WATCH: A One-Two to the Brain." *Discover* (Nov. 1994) 36-37.

Roach, Mary, "Advice from the World's Biggest Weight Experts: Their Gain Can Be Your Loss." *Health* (March/April 1993) 62-72.
(Describes the traditional, low-fat diet of Japanese sumo wrestlers.)

Rosenberg, Steven A., "Adoptive Immunotherapy for Cancer." *Scientific American* (May 1990) 62-69.

Scientific American, Special Issue: "Life, Death and the Immune System." (Sept. 1993) entire issue.

Scrimshaw, Nevin S., "Iron Deficiency." *Scientific American* (Oct., 1991) 46-52.
(Explains how vegetarian diets lead to anemia, lethargy and reduced IQ in children.)

Serra-Majem, Lluis *et al,* "How could changes in diet explain changes in coronary heart disease mortality in Spain? The Spanish paradox." *American Journal of Clinical Nutrition* (1995) 1351S-9S.

Shaper, A. G. *et al,* "Cardiovascular studies in the Samburu tribe of Northern Kenya." *American Heart Journal* Vol. 63 No. 4 (April 1962) 437-442.

Shepard, Paul, "A Post-Historic Primitivism." For "The Wilderness Condition: *Realia* Conference on Environment and Civilization" Estes Park, CO (August 17-23, 1989).
(Hunter-gatherer philosophy for the modern man.)

Speth, John D., "Early Hominid Hunting and Scavenging: The Role of Meat as an Energy Source." *Journal of Human Evolution* Vol. 18 (1989) 329-343.
(Attempts to calculate the amount of meat and fat required for hominid survival.)

Stahl, Ann Brower, "Hominid Dietary Selection Before Fire." *Current Anthropology* Vol. 25, No. 2 (April 1984) 151-68.
(Explains the constraints on human diet without fire.)

Stipp, David, "The Way We Were: Our Prehistoric Past Casts Ills in New Light, Some Scientists Say." *The Wall Street Journal* (Wednesday, May 24, 1995) 1 & A6, Col. 1.

United Press International, "Anthropologist: Eat like a caveman and live to 100." *The San Diego Union* (Saturday, Oct. 14, 1989) C-6.

Wallis, Michael, "ANTHROPOLOGIST VAUGHN BRYANT LOST 30 POUNDS (BUT NOT HIS HEALTH) EATING WHAT THE CAVE DWELLERS ATE." *People* (Feb. 19, 1979) 103-4.

Washington, Harriet, "The back to the future diet; healthy diet habits of traditional cultures." *Harvard Health Letter* (June 1994) 6.

Wurtman, Richard J. and Judith J., "Carbohydrates and Depression." *Scientific American* (Jan. 1989) 68-75.
(Explains the role of complex carbohydrates in mood swings.)

Zane, Frank, Bodybuilding Advisory: Train with Zane "Eating for muscular definition." *Muscle & Fitness* (Dec. 1994) 226.

Zvelebil, Marek, "Postglacial Foraging in the Forests of Europe." *Scientific American* (May 1986) 104-115.
(Documents the Neolithic Revolution in Europe.)

BOOKS

Ardrey, Robert, *African Genesis.* New York: Antheneum, 1961.

Ardrey, Robert, *The Hunting Hypothesis*. New York: Atheneum, 1976.

Atkins, Robert C., *Dr. Atkins' Diet Revolution*. New York: Bantam Books, 1972.

Atkins, Robert C., *Dr. Atkins' Super-Energy Diet*. New York: Bantam Books, 1977.

Bruce, Scott and Bill Crawford, *Cerealizing America: The Unsweetened Story of American Breakfast Cereal.* Boston & London: Faber and Faber, 1995.
(Details the history of breakfast cereal in America with a brilliant section on the history of Dr. John Harvey Kellogg as told in the feature film The Road to Wellville.*)*

Bryant, Vaughn, "The Paleolithic Health Club." *1995 Yearbook of Science and the Future*. Chicago: Encyclopedia Britannica, Inc. (1994) 114-133.

Budiansky, Stephen, *The Covenant of the Wild: Why Animals Chose Domestication*. New York: William Morrow & Co., Inc., 1992.
(Explains the role of neoteny in the Neolithic Revolution and how it was as much a biological as a technological revolution.)

Campbell, Ada Marie, Marjorie Porter Penfield and Ruth M. Griswold, *The Experimental Study of Food*. 2nd ed. Boston: Houghton Mifflin Co., 1979.

Chatwin, Bruce, *The Songlines*. New York: Viking, 1987.
(Talks about the religion of Australian Aborigines in particular and hunter-gathering in general.)

Cohen, Mark Nathan, *The Food Crisis in Prehistory: Overpopulation and the Origins of Agriculture*. New Haven: Yale University Press, 1977.
(How environmental changes led man to seek new food sources.)

_____, *Health and the Rise of Civilization*. New Haven: Yale University Press, 1993.
(How man's new food sources produced new diseases.)

Corballis, Michael L., *The Lopsided Ape: Evolution of the Generative Mind.* Oxford:
Oxford University Press, 1991.
(Talks about how the difference in left- and right-brain size affected the evolution of human behavior.)

Crawford, Michael and Sheilagh, *What We Eat Today: The Food Manipulators vs. the People.*
New York: Stein & Day, 1972.

Desowitz, Robert S., *New Guinea Tape Worms and Jewish Grandmothers: Tales of Parasites and People.* New York, Avon Books, 1981

Diamond, Jared, *The Third Chimpanzee: The Evolution and Future of the Human Animal.*
New York: Harper Perennial, 1992.

DiPasquale, Dr. Mauro, *The Anabolic Diet.* Optimum Training Systems, 1995.
(Low-carbohydrate diet used by bodybuilders and professional wrestlers.)

Eades, Michael R., M.D., *Thin So Fast.* New York, New York: Warner Books, 1989.

Eades, Michael R., M.D. and Mary Dan, M.D., *Protein Power.* New York: Bantam, 1995.
(Highly recommended. Explains how low-carbohydrate diets work focusing especially on insulin resistance. Excellent chapters on ancient diet and cholesterol metabolism.)

Eaton, S. Boyd, Marjorie Shostak and Melvin Konner,
   The Paleolithic Prescription. New York:
   Harper & Row, 1988.
(Arose from the landmark 1985 article in The New
England Journal of Medicine. *Constitutes a very
conservative approach to Paleolithic Nutrition.)*

Farb, Peter and George Armelagos, *Consuming
   Passions: The Anthropology of Eating*.
   Boston: Houghton Mifflin Co., 1980.

Fieldhouse, Paul, *Food & Nutrition: Customs &
   Culture*. London: Croom Helm, 1986.

Gare, Fran and Helen Monica, *Dr. Atkins' Diet
   Cookbook*. New York: Bantam Books, 1974.

Gasset, Jose Ortega y, *Meditations on Hunting*.
   New York: Charles Scribner Sons, 1972.
*(Modern   ruminations   on   hunter-gatherer
philosophy.)*

Harris, Marvin and Eric B. Ross, *FOOD and
   Evolution*. Philadelphia: Temple University
   Press, 1987.

Harris, Marvin, *Cannibals and Kings: The Origins of
   Cultures*. New York: Random House, 1977.
*(The story of how the needs of crop species forced
man to become civilized.)*

Harris, Marvin, *Good to Eat: Riddles of Food &
   Culture*. New York: Simon & Schuster, 1985.

Hunter, Beatrice Trum, *The Great Nutrition
    Robbery*. New York: Charles Scribner's Sons,
    1978.

Lee, Richard B. and Irven Devore, *Man the Hunter*.
    Chicago: Aldine Publishing Co., 1968.

Oelschlager, Max, *The Idea of Wilderness*.
    New Haven and London: Yale University
    Press, 1991.
*(How our agricultural view of nature affects the
environment.)*

Sauer, Carl O., *Seeds, Spades, Hearths & Herds:
    The Domestication of Animals and
    Foodstuffs*. 2nd ed., Cambridge:
    The MIT Press, 1969.

Sieden, Lloyd Steven, *Buckminster Fuller's Universe:
    An Appreciation*. New York & London:
    Plenum Press, 1989, 367-68.

Shepard, Paul, *The Tender Carnivore and the Sacred
    Game*. New York: Charles Scribner and Sons,
    1973.
*(A manifesto concerning how agriculture and
neoteny conspire to oppress humans and destroy the
environment.)*

Stefansson, Vilhjalmur, *Cancer: Disease of Civilization.* New York: Hill and Wang, 1960. *(Documents the unsuccessful search for cancer and other autoimmune disorders among hunter-gatherers.)*

_____, *Hunters of the Great North.* New York: Harcourt, Brace & Co., 1922.

_____, *The Fat of the Land* (originally, *Not By Bread Alone,* 1946). New York: Macmillan, 1956. *(The definitive, and only, book on pemmican.)*

Tannahill, Reay, *Food In History.* New York: Stein & Day, 1973. *(Talks about the origins of the foods we eat today.)*

Winterhalder, Bruce and Eric Alden Smith, *Hunter-Gatherer Foraging Strategies: Ethnographic and Archeological Analyses.* Chicago: Univ. of Chicago Press, 1981.

Wright, Robert, *The Moral Animal: Why We Are the Way We Are: The New Science of Evolutionary Psychology.* New York: Pantheon Books, 1994. *(Discusses how our hunting and gathering instincts are the evolutionary basis of our morality.)*

The Authors

Ray Audette is a falconer in Dallas, Texas. When not hunting or gathering, Ray lectures, consults and writes about Paleolithic Nutrition. He is also professionally engaged in publishing, computer marketing, advertising and photography. Ray received a Bachelor of Science degree from The University of Texas in 1975. He is actively involved in the Texas Hawking Association and Mensa and is a Board Member of the Dallas Philosophers' Forum.

Troy Gilchrist has been Ray's assistant since graduating with a B. A. degree in Philosophy from the University of North Texas in 1994. He is a certified massage therapist and a professional guitarist and songwriter.